Herb Remedy Recipes for Beginners

Using and Making Herbal Remedies

Carolyn Gibson
Family Herbalist, LMT MTI

DISCLAIMER

This information in this book is for educational purposes only and is not meant to be used as medical advice. This book is not intended to diagnose, prescribe, or treat any disease, illness or injury to the body. The author, the publisher and the distributor does not accept any responsibility for such use. Always consult your physician or medical professional for disease, illness or injury.

To err is human. Every attempt has been made to make sure all information is accurate. The author and publisher are not responsible for errors.

ACKNOWLEDGMENTS

I have relied on information from many herbalists and my own experience. David Hoffman's The Herbal Handbook and his book, Medical Herbalism; the writing, and teaching of Dr. John Christopher and David Christopher at the School of Natural Healing, the books and teachings of Rosemary Gladstar, Rosalee de la Foret from Herb Mentor and so many more. I was blessed to have Odena Brannam, considered the grandmother of herbs in Texas to mentor me in the study of herbs and taught me to go beyond herbal teas and to make my first herbal medicine. I find The American Botanical Council to be an invaluable source of information and encourage everyone to join and support their work. I have been studying and practicing herbs since the early 1970's and I will never know enough to quit studying and learning.

I praise and honor God the Father and thank him for his gifts.

Honor God the Father and not His creations.

RECIPE INDEX

Carolyn Gibson

REMEDY INDEX

Carolyn Gibson

1 Introduction

Herbs are healing plants given to us by God for our use, however they are not magic potions nor miracle drugs. They are our first recourse for healing but not the only recourse. They are a first step, if you are not healing see your medical professional. God also gave us doctors, hospitals, and real drugs, which can be overused, but are sometimes necessary. This is not a religion. You can use herbal remedies and rely on your medical professional when necessary.

Herb Remedy Recipes is meant to be a beginner's guide to making herb oils, salves and tinctures for everyday common ailments. I have tried to recommend some already made products, for those times that sickness strikes and you have not had opportunity to make that particular remedy. And believe me, it is impossible to make everything you will need.

This is not a book for every possible ailment and does not include every possible remedy. This book includes a variety remedies for you to try. There are countless remedies for the same ailment recommended and used by many herbalists. This book is for those who do not have any serious health issues, who are mostly adults.

Not every herb will work for every person.

As important as herbs are, diet and exercise are even more important. Of course over the years "what is a good diet" is constantly changing.

Your body is like a machine, the muscles are like pulleys which must be pulled and released to work, the circulation system is like the fluid in a hydraulic system, which doesn't work without adequate fluid and doesn't work at all without the pulleys pumping the pumps, and good fats and oils to lubricate the whole system.

Research is now showing the importance of good bacteria in your gut. The right bacteria not only effects your digestive system, but also your immune system, your nervous system, your emotions and moods and all the other systems of the body.

You may find as you begin your herbal journey illness may strike before you have began making your herbal remedies. If you are the healer in your family, you may be in no condition to begin making herbal remedies. I have listed herbal preparations that are already made and available at health food stores. There are a few that can be made in a few minutes. Many of the herbal remedies must be made in advance and stored until you need them.

Herbs are listed may be as close as your grocery store, and others may be at your health food store, or you may have to purchase them online.

I will include page numbers so that you can find the recipes quickly.

Remember: Herbal Remedies are not a religion, they are not magic potions or miracles in a bottle. Herbs are your first resource, if they are not working use the drugs available at your drug store or seek medical attention.

Warning: Herbs can become an obsession. You may quickly run out of space to plant the many herbs you have read about and eagerly searched for and bought. Herb books and magazines may overspill your shelves.

You may find herb tinctures macerating, cluttering up your kitchen, herb syrups filling up your refrigerator, prepared remedies overcrowding your pantry, and bunches of herbs drying all over your house. If you do not become fanatical about labeling your remedies, I promise, you will forget what is what.

This will be your journey and your pursuit to determine which herbs work for you and your family. As you experience the benefits from these simple remedies I hope you may be inspired to learn more and more and find that you have a healer growing inside of you.

This book is divided into 6 categories of illness:
- Colds, Flu, Allergies and Fever
- First Aid
- Pain
- Sleep and Stress
- Tummy Alert
- Women's Concerns

As you read each chapter the remedy that you need to make will be in italics and bold with the page number for making it. Each chapter is then divided into symptoms with page numbers to quickly find your remedy.

Next will be a chapter on the basics of making herbal remedies with recipes or formulas. There will be remedies repeated in the book. Some ailments apply to more than one category, example: ear ache is listed in both the chapter on colds, flu and allergies, and also under pain. I want to make sure you can find it.

The 2 remaining chapters will be additional recipes and a description of some of the herbs mentioned in this book.

Many of the remedies must be made 2-6 weeks in advance. All dosages are for healthy adults.

Much of this information will be on my website, www.FamilyGuidetoHerbs.com and I will be adding more information, more recipes and videos. Visit me for herbal kits, herbs and supplies.

Caution: Natural does not mean safe for everyone. Always check with your medical professional if you have serious health conditions or an auto immune system disorder. If you are pregnant or nursing check with your health care professional before taking any herbs.

General Cautions:
Hops: Do not use if you have a family history of breast cancer.
Kava Kava: Do not use if you are pregnant or nursing, have a liver disorder, use prescriptions or take acetaminophen, or drink excessive alcohol.
Passionflower: Do not take if pregnant or nursing, may interfere with blood thinning medicine.
St. John's Wort: Potential to interact with prescription medicine. Safety in pregnancy has not been established.
Garlic: Discontinue use 10 days before surgery, do not eat over 4 cloves a day if on anticoagulant medication, can

interfere with medicine for HIV.

Ginger: Do not take excessive amounts with blood thinners, may cause heartburn.

Licorice Root: Long term use may deplete the body's potassium and cause water retention which will lead to high blood pressure. Use a DGL version. Those with high blood pressure, kidney or heart problems, taking blood thinners, or blood pressure medicine should use caution with licorice root. Not recommended for those that are pregnant or breast feeding.

Peppermint: Use with caution if you have GERD, or hiatal hernia do not give to children under 3.

Use caution with all the anti- spasmodic herbs if you are on medication for insomnia or anxiety as these may increase their effects.

Use caution with all anti-spasmodic herbs before driving or operating machinery until you see how they affect you personally, could cause drowsiness.

2 Colds, Flu, Allergies and Fevers

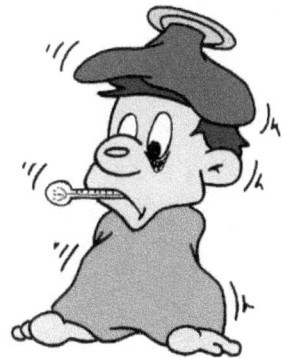

This book will start off with the most common ailment that affects us all: Colds, Allergies the Flu and Fevers. You can determine if it is a cold or flu by how suddenly it appears and how intense. You may find yourself trying to treat a cold when it is an allergy.

When choosing herbs for a cough or sore throat, it is more than deciding which herb is for a cough or sore throat. What kind of cough? Is your throat hot and swollen or dry and itchy? Do you have runny mucus, or do you have thick, stuck mucus? There are even different types of fever which are treated differently. Who knew? Who came up with that?

Check out your symptoms and then go the page number for that symptom.

Remember all dosages are for adults.

SYMPTOMS

SYMPTOMS MEAN THE IMMUNE SYSTEM IS DOING ITS JOB.

God made your body to fight off infections and other toxic invasions.

Symptoms that are so uncomfortable and maybe even painful are the immune system doing its job.

In his love and mercy, God also gave us plants or herbs to help us deal with these symptoms while working with the immune system.

While drug company solutions may lessen the symptoms and seem to work quicker, they may work against God's plan for the immune system and cause unpleasant or even dangerous side effects.

Whether it be a sore throat, coughing, runny nose, stopped up nose, fever, etc., there are herbal ways to deal with these symptoms that will support your immune system while relieving your symptoms.

A cough with mucus is treated differently than a cough without mucus. A hot and swollen throat is treated differently than a dry itchy throat. There are even differences in how to treat a fever.

SYMPTOMS: COLD, FLU OR ALLERGY

Cold
Symptoms begin 2-3 days, lasts 1-2 weeks

Stuffy or runny nose
Mild fever possible
Mild aches
Mild chills
Sore throat
Fatigue
Headache
Sinus drainage
Mild cough
Watery eyes
Ear Congestion
Sneezing

Flu
Symptoms begin within 2-3 hours, last 1-2 weeks

Body aches or pain you can feel all the way to the bones
Stuffy or runny nose
Fever 100 ºF or higher
Intense chills
Sore throat
Fatigue lasting weeks after recovery
Extreme exhaustion
Headaches
Diarrhea and vomiting
Cough
Watery eyes with fever
Sneezing

Allergy symptoms are very similar, the main symptoms that are different are eyes that are itchy, watery, burning and swollen. You will not have the ache or body pain. An allergy will lasts as long as the allergens are around while the cold or flu will last only a week or two.

FIRST SIGN OF COLD OR FLU

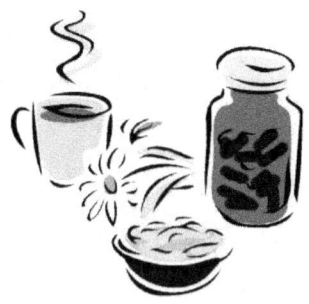

Elderberry

Elderberry Syrup pg. 107: 1-2 tablespoons per hour or at least several times a day
Or *Elderberry Tincture pg. 101:* 30-60 drops (1/4 to ½ teaspoon) every hour or least several times a day
With:
Echinacea Tincture pg. 99: 30-60 drops (1/4 to ½ teaspoon) every hour or at least several times a day
Caution: If you have an auto immune disorder, check with your health care professional before taking Echinacea.

Or: Ginger

Ginger Tea with honey, optional with a pinch cayenne pepper
Iced Ginger Tea (Ginger ale)
Ginger Oxymel pg. 121

Or: Garlic

Use lots of Garlic
Garlic honey: 1 spoonful throughout the day
Garlic butter on bread throughout the day
Garlic Cider Vinegar pg. 137: 1 tablespoon every hour or several times a day

ELDERBERRY VS TAMIFLU

The Sambucol Elderberry Syrup Study Showed:
- Studies showed it decreased the flu symptoms by 3-4 days
- Dosage: 2-4 teaspoons ever hour or up to 1 tablespoon 4 times a day
- Side effects: none

So safe you can use Elderberry syrup on your pancakes.

Source: National Geographic Guide to Medicinal Herbs and The Herbal Drugstore.

Tamiflu:

Requires a prescription
Decreases the flu by 1 day
Side effects: Mild to moderate nausea and vomiting, diarrhea, stomach pain.

Sources: Tamiflu.com and TV commercials, WebMD

Elderberry syrups are available at most drug stores and health food stores. The brand Sambucal is the brand used in the studies.

You can find Elderberry Extracts or Syrups at most health food stores or online.

Elderberry Syrup Recipe: pg. 107

Despite your preventive efforts you become sick:

If you have been under stress, overworked, and worried the body will demand rest and relief. If that means getting sick, or an injury, that is the price you pay.

If you have been overindulging in the wrong foods and drinks, which creates mucus, the body will cleanse itself.

At this point all you can do is to treat the symptoms in a way that will help the body do its job.

SORE THROAT: HOT AND SWOLLEN

Astringent herbs that tighten and tone the mucosal membrane: Sage or Yarrow

Anodyne herbs that dull or numb the pain: Echinacea Root or Clove

Only Echinacea roots or seeds are for dulling the pain, the upper portions will not dull or numb the pain.

Sage Tea:
1 teaspoon of sage leaves
1 cup of boiling water
Honey to taste
Lemon juice to taste
Pour boiling water over sage leaves, cover and steep for 10 minutes. Strain and add honey and lemon juice to taste. Sip as a tea.

Use as a gargle or use to spray the throat.

Essential oil of clove can be mixed into the honey prior to mixing with tea to use as a gargle or a throat spray.

Sage Tincture pg. 102 and Echinacea Root Tincture pg. 99 **as a gargle or a throat spray**

Combine Sage and Echinacea Root Tincture 2 ½ ml (½ teaspoon) of Sage Tincture and 2 ½ ml (½ teaspoon) of Echinacea Root Tincture to 1 cup of warm water and gargle

Add a combination of Sage and Echinacea tincture to a spray bottle and spray the throat 3 times a day or as needed.

Clinical study involving 154 patients with acute sore throats found that a Sage and Echinacea Root throat spray to be as effective as a Chlorhexidine/Lidocaine Throat Spray.

Source: National Geographic Guide to Medicinal Herbs

Caution: Do not use Sage alcohol preparation for more than 2 weeks.

Use Lozenges or throat sprays that contain Sage and Echinacea Root.

Try Gaia Sage and Aloe Shield Spray or Lozenges at Amazon.com or MountainRoseHerbs.com or a local health food store.

IS IT STREP THROAT?

Strep throat is a bacterial infection, while colds and flu are viral infections, and only a test by the doctor can confirm if the infection is strep throat.

Symptoms

Sudden throat pain without coughing, sneezing, and other symptoms of a cold.
Difficulty or pain with swallowing.
Fever of 101°F. or more. A lower fever may indicate a viral infection instead of strep.
Red and swollen tonsils.
White or yellow spots or a coating on the throat and tonsils.
Bright red spots on the throat.
Dark red spots back on the roof of the mouth.
Swollen, tender lymph glands in the neck.
Fever.
Headache.
Rash.
Stomach ache and sometimes vomiting in young children.
Fatigue.

If a rough rash develops and spreads over the neck and chest and then to rest of the body this could indicate scarlet fever.

If you develop the below symptoms 1-2 weeks after the strep infection, you may have rheumatic fever see a doctor.

Weakness
Shortness of breath
Joint pain
Raised red rash or lumps under the skin
Uncontrolled, jerking movements of the arms or legs

TREATING STREP THROAT OR TONSILLITIS

Soothe the sore throat with the same treatments for a hot and swollen sore throat. Pg. 21

Fight the infection with Garlic and Honey.
Source: Fawn and John Christopher, School of Natural Healing.

Garlic: When using garlic as an antibiotic or antimicrobial mince the garlic and let it set 10-15 minutes. The garlic cells must be ruptured to release two separate chemicals of the garlic, alliin and alliinase which then form a new compound called allicin.

Chop or mince 3-4 cloves of garlic. Let set 10-15 minutes. Add 1 tablespoon of honey and 1/8 – 1/4 teaspoon of cayenne pepper. Take this ever hour all day.

Other options:

3 parts Mullein and 1 part Lobelia
Rub on the throat as a salve, or prepare a tea and make a fomentation; drink as a tea or take as a tincture. Prepare salve according to salve and ointment instructions on page 113 using 3 parts Mullein and 1 part Lobelia.

Tea to drink: Pour 1 cup of boiling water over 1 teaspoon of the herb mixture. Cover and steep 10 minutes. Strain, may be reheated. Add honey to taste. Drink ½ cup 3 times a day.

Mullein/Lobelia Tincture take 5 ml (1 teaspoon) 3 times a day or 2.5 ml to 5 ml (1/2- 1 teaspoon) ever hour. Prepare according to Tincture instruction of page 91 using 3 parts Mullein and 1 part Lobelia.

Fomentation: Make a strong tea: Pour 2 cups of boiling water over 2 tablespoons of herb mixture. Cover and steep 10 minutes. Strain. Dip a natural cloth such as cotton, wool or linen and into the tea. Wring out and place on throat. Cover with a plastic wrap and then cover with dry cloth. Leave on overnight. Continue until throat is healed. The plastic wrap forces the tea into the skin and off your clothes. The dry cloth creates heat opening the pores of the skin to drive the herbs further in.

Take *Echinacea Tincture Pg. 99:* 1 dropper full ever hour (1/4 teaspoon)

SORE THROAT; DRY AND ITCHY, NO MUCUS

Slipping and sliding: soothe, moisten and protect the throat with demulcent herbs; herbs that are rich in mucilage (slippery).

Use Anti-Spasmodic herbs to stop the cough reflex causing more irritation and so you can get some sleep.

Demulcent Herbs:

Licorice Root

Marshmallow

Slippery Elm

Honey

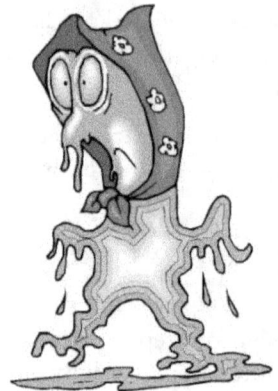

Throat lozenges or teas that contain at least one of these demulcent herbs, Licorice Root, Marshmallow, Plantain, Slippery Elm and honey.

Project: Slippery Elm Throat Soothers pg. 122

Try these at your local health food store, St. Claire's Throat Soothers, Thayer's Slippery Elm Lozenges, and Throat Coat Tea by Traditional Medicines.

Licorice Root Tea

Since this is a root it must be simmered 15-20 minutes to draw out its properties.

Licorice root is extremely sweet so other herbs are usually added to it. Use 2 parts Licorice and then add 1 part of these other optional herbs, Echinacea root, Cinnamon, Ginger root, Marshmallow, Wild Cherry Bark, or Slippery Elm. After it has simmered you could add herbs such as Peppermint, Sage, Plantain, etc and let steep for 5-10 minutes. Add honey to taste.

Long term use of Licorice Root may cause water retention, which will then cause high blood pressure.

Anti- Spasmodic Herbs: Cough Suppressant

California Poppy for daytime use and safe for children. Adults start with 30 drops, (1/4 teaspoon) if that does not work take more until coughing stops.

Lobelia Tincture: Lobelia is a powerful herb you take very little of. Start with a few drops, wait 10 minutes and then add more if needed. Too much will cause vomiting. Depending on the strength and your sensitivity you may need as much as ¼ teaspoon.

Lobelia not recommend for pregnant or nursing.

Valerian Tincture: Great muscle relaxer. Adults start with 30 drops (1/4 teaspoon) and if that does not work try more until coughing does stop. Valerian is considered a sedative, so for some, it is best taken at night. I take it during the day and it is not a problem. Valerian may have the opposite effect on some people and wire them up instead of sedating them.

Wild Cherry Bark Cough Syrup: Look out for imitations on the market. Make sure it is Wild Cherry Bark and not cherry flavored.

Honey by itself can help with coughs.

SWOLLEN GLANDS

The premiere herbs of choice for swollen glands are 3 parts **Mullein** to 1 part **Lobelia.**

Take internally as a tincture, externally as a poultice, or rub on as a salve, or rub the tincture into the area.

Mullein/Lobelia Tea to drink: Pour 1 cup of boiling water over 1 teaspoon of the herb mixture. Cover and steep 10 minutes. Strain. May be reheated. Add honey to taste. Drink ½ cup 3 times a day.

Mullein/Lobelia Tincture take 1 teaspoon 3 times a day or 1/2-1 teaspoon ever hour. Apply the Mullein/Lobelia tincture externally to the throat.

Fomentation: Make a Mullein/Lobelia strong tea: Pour 2 cups of boiling water over 2 tablespoons of herb mixture. Cover and steep 10 minutes. Strain. Dip a natural cloth such as cotton, wool or linen and into the tea. Wring out and place on throat. Cover with a plastic wrap and then cover with dry cloth. Leave on overnight. Continue until throat is healed. The plastic wrap forces the tea into the skin and off your clothes. The dry cloth creates heat, opening the pores of the skin to drive the herbs further in.

Prepare a salve according to instructions on page 113 using 3 parts Mullein to 1 part Lobelia.

Prepare tincture according to instructions on pg. 91 using 3 parts Mullein to 1 part Lobelia.

Add *Echinacea Root Tincture* pg. 99 as a throat spray or take internally.

MUCUS

One of the first symptoms of the cold, flu or allergies is mucus. And we naturally will want to stop it. Herb books and herbalist call excess mucus, catarrh or catarrhal inflammation.

We need mucus. It is a part of our immune system. All parts of our bodies are lined with mucus membranes which produce mucus. Mucus contains our antibodies. Mucus is that slimy, slippery stuff that contains antibodies to every organism that has ever attacked our bodies. Mucus's mission in our life is to stop invading pathogens and irritants from reaching our mucus membranes.

Although unpleasant, stopping the mucus may lengthen the duration of your illness, and worse may lead to infections in the sinus or lungs.

But this does not mean we need to suffer needlessly.

Good Mucus: thin, clear and running.

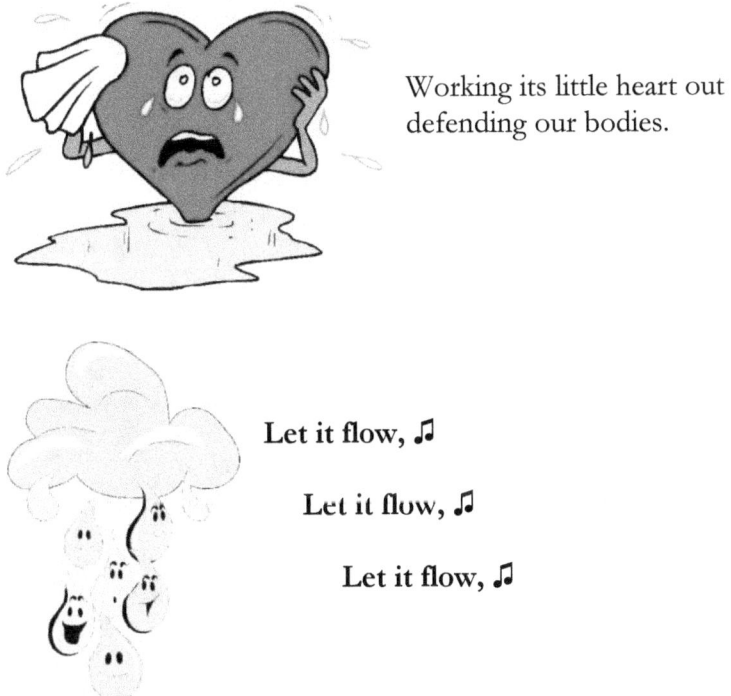

Working its little heart out defending our bodies.

Let it flow, ♫

Let it flow, ♫

Let it flow, ♫

Keep it flowing with warm spicy foods and plenty of liquids.

RUNNY NOSE

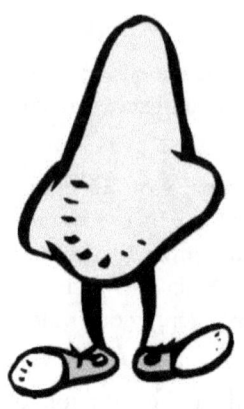

The Immune System
Doing its job

Keep it flowing with these
stimulating herbs

Ginger tea with a pinch of cayenne pepper and honey,

Ginger Oxymel pg. 121

Or try chewing on a piece of Ginger, or Ginger Candy

Hot Chicken Soup or Tortilla Soup steeped with Thyme pg. 139-140

Garlic Butter or Honey pg. 136

Garlic Cider Vinegar pg.137

Peppermint or Spearmint tea with honey.

Nose Irrigation: Salt water, 1 cup of water with 1/4-1/2 teaspoon of salt, either a Neti Pot, or I use a syringe

Tincture: 3 parts Mullein with 1 part Lobelia: Prepare according to instructions on pg. 91.

5 ml (1 teaspoon) throughout the day

Steam Inhalation with or without the addition of essential oils of Peppermint or Eucalyptus

STOPPING THE DRIP

Amazingly all that you do to keep the mucus flowing will eventually stop the flow.

If you cannot wait for your body's natural cleansing, and your drippy nose is just off the charts and you really need to stop it because of work and other obligations there is relief in sight.

When your tissues are swollen, inflamed and running like a river you need anti-catarrhal herbs that acts as an astringent and an anti-inflammatory.

Anti-Catarrhal: Herbs that reduce excessive mucus

Elderflowers, not the berries, combined with Peppermint. Peppermint is also added to offset the possibility of the Elderflowers causing nausea.

Optional: add these additional herbs:
Yarrow
Echinacea

Use this combination as a tea or tincture.

Best results is to do a nasal wash several times a day with either a neti pot or spray bottle or a syringe combining 1/4 teaspoon of salt with 8 oz. of an herbal tea.

If the runny nose is due to an allergy try Nettle, Eyebright, or Ragweed extracts capsules. Ragweed would be the most effective but the hardest to find.

WHEN GOOD MUCUS GOES BAD

Bad Mucus:

Clear mucus that gets congested

White, seems stuck

Green and yellow indicates infection

STOPPED UP NOSE: STUCK MUCUS

That familiar remedy from your childhood, get out the Vicks. Vicks is basically petroleum jelly with menthol. Menthol comes from Peppermint and other mint species. Spread on your throat, chest and on the cheek bones. Caution: Do not get near the eyes.

Or

Add essential oil of Peppermint or Eucalyptus to some lotion or oil and use the same as Vicks. If your nose is too clogged up for the Peppermint Oil to penetrate or if your skin is hyper sensitive to the oil:

Mix 3 drops of essential oil of Peppermint to 2 tablespoons of honey. Place a pea size of this mixture on the back of the tongue. The molecules of the essential oil of Peppermint can go behind the pharynx into the nasal cavities as a decongestant.

Optional: Mix equal amounts of essential oils of Peppermint, Eucalyptus and Lavender and replace this mixture for the essential oil of Peppermint.

Ephedra is the supreme herb for decongesting. I have not found another herb that works as well. Due to the misuse of Ephedra by the "lose weight" marketers, Ephedra has been taken off the market. The only way to get this herb is to grow it yourself.

Ephedra and any pharmaceutical decongestant are stimulants and will keep you awake at night.

Breathing in steam will help to break up the congestion. This can be done by drinking a hot tea such as Peppermint tea or other herbal tea. Bringing water to a boil, add herbs such as Thyme, Peppermint, or Sage, remove from the heat and breathe in the steam. If no herbs are available use plain steam. Take a hot shower or bath.

Use a humidifier.

Nose Wash: Mix 8 oz. of herbal tea or water with 1/4 teaspoon of salt, use a neti pot, spray bottle or syringe to cleanse the nose. If your nose is so stopped up that a nose wash will not penetrate, do a steam inhalation first.

Note: Fresh or dried herbs can be used, or tinctures of the herbs.

Caution on using the essential oils of these herbs; only use a few drops.

DRY NOSE

Dry and irritated, maybe a bleeding nose, mucus is dry causing picking of your nose to get it out.

Hydration: plenty of liquids and good fats in your diet.

Demulcent Herbs:
Marshmallow Root
Mullein
Licorice Root
Slippery elm

Make a tea from one of the above herbs straining well and let cool.

Most herbal teas are made by either simmering the roots or steeping leaves, Marshmallow Root is not steeped or simmered. It is soaked in cold water for at least 4 hours.

Fill a cup 1/4 the way with Marshmallow Root or 1 teaspoon of powdered Marshmallow Root, add water and let set for 4 hours or overnight. This will make a thick liquid.

Licorice Root or Slippery Elm Bark tea:
Add 1 teaspoon of the chopped Licorice root or Slippery Elm Bark, or ½ teaspoon of the powder to 1 cup of boiling water and simmer 15-20 minutes. Remove from heat and cool.

Mullein Leaf Tea:
Add 1 teaspoon of chopped leaves to 8 oz. of boiling water. Remove from heat, cover and steep 10-15 minutes. Let cool.
Strain any of these well.

You can either dip a cotton ball into these teas and place in your nose for 10-20 minutes (be sure and leave enough cotton ball hanging out to remove the cotton ball) or use as a nasal rinse adding 1/4 teaspoon of salt to 8 oz. of tea.

Rub an oil or herb infused oil, pg. 110 or herbal salve inside your nose. Pg. 113.

Long term use of Licorice Root may cause water retention, which will then cause high blood pressure.

SIGNS OF INFECTION

Green Mucus with fever or sinus pain.

Infections can be bacteria, viral, or fungal.

Herbs are anti-microbial, not anti-biotic so therefore fight all three kinds of infection.

Garlic: When using garlic as an antibiotic or antimicrobial mince the garlic and let it set 10-15 minutes. The garlic cells must be ruptured to release two separate chemicals of the garlic, alliin and alliinase which then form a new compound called allicin.

3 cloves of garlic minced, let set for 10-15 minutes, add honey and eat throughout the day, according to how your stomach can handle it. Pg. 136.

Or

Garlic minced, let set out 10-15 minutes add butter or olive oil and eat throughout the day according to how your stomach can handle it. Pg. 136.

Optional:

Echinacea Tincture pg. 99: Take 1 teaspoon ever 2 hours or use as a throat spray.

Or

Golden Seal: This herb must touch the area affected. Either make a tea, or use a tincture in a nose wash with 1/4 teaspoon of salt to 8 oz. of water.

If you do not see improvement see your doctor.

COUGHS WITH MUCUS

Cough, Cough, Get it out! Get it out!

The body is trying to eliminate either excess mucus or other irritants. Keeping the mucus or irritants in the lungs can lead to infection or pneumonia. At the very least prolong your illness.

Only take a suppressant (anti-spasmodic) so that you can sleep at night or for a few hours for work, church, etc.

Choose syrups or lozenges that say Expectorant. Expectorants do not make you cough. An expectorant thins the mucus so that it become easier to cough up.

Mission: Help cough up the mucus by keeping it thin and running with stimulating herbs and aromatic herbs.

Mustard, Horseradish, Onions, Garlic, Ginger, Other Spicy Foods.

Garlic Cider Vinegar pg. 137

Ginger Oxymel pg. 121

Peppermint Tea, Salve or essential oil of Peppermint with honey, pg. 30
Ginger Tea, Ginger Candy
Cayenne Pepper Tea
Hot Salsa with corn tortillas or chips, not flour
Mullein
Facial Steams, Hot showers, hot baths

Garlic Syrup, Ginger Syrup, Ginger Candy Crystallized Ginger
Root it Away Syrup from Terra Firma Botanicals
Cough Care from Mountain Rose Herbs

DRY, HACKING COUGHS, NO MUCUS

Now is when you need a suppressant, otherwise known as an anti-spasmodic.

Do not use expectorant herbs in this dry condition. This will only make matters worse.

Choose Syrups, Lozenges or Extracts with at least one these herbs:

Moisturize with demulcent herbs:
Licorice Root
Marshmallow Root
Slippery Elm
Honey

Anti-Spasmodic Herbs to stop the cough since there is nothing to cough up:

California Poppy for daytime use and safe for children. Adults start with 30 drops (1/4 teaspoon) if that does not work take more until coughing stops.

Lobelia Tincture: Lobelia is a powerful herb you take very little of. Start with a few drops, wait 10 minutes and then add more if needed. Depending on the strength of the tincture and your sensitivity you may need as much as a ¼ teaspoon. Too much will cause nausea or vomiting. Prepare Lobelia according to instructions for making tincture. Pg. 91

Valerian Extract or Tincture: Great muscle relaxer. Adults start with 30 drops (1/4 teaspoon) and if that does not work try more until coughing does stop. Valerian is considered a sedative, so for some people it is best taken at night. Valerian may have the opposite effect on some people and wire them up instead of sedating them.

Wild Cherry Bark: when buying Wild Cherry Cough Syrup beware of imitations. Make sure the bottle says Wild Cherry Bark and not cherry flavored.

I like to use *the Slippery Elm Throat Soothers* pg. 122 to soothe my cough and use the Lobelia tincture as the anti spasmodic.

If all this looks familiar it is the same as for a dry itchy throat.

Long term use of Licorice Root may cause water retention, which will then cause high blood pressure. Lobelia not recommended if pregnant or nursing.

UNPRODUCTIVE COUGH: DRIED UP MUCUS THAT NEEDS TO COME UP

You are coughing up some mucus, but it feels like there is more and you just cannot get it up. You may even have a yellow tongue.

Mission: Moisten and thin the mucus with moistening, expectorant herbs. You may need some anti-microbial herbs.

Choose lozenges, syrups, or tinctures that contain at least one herb from each of these categories.

Demulcent (moistening herbs):
Licorice Root
Marshmallow Root
Mullein
Slippery Elm
Honey

Expectorant Herbs: thins the mucus:
Ginger
Garlic
Onions
Hyssop
Licorice Root
Mullein
White horehound

Anti-Microbial
Clove
Echinacea
Goldenseal
Licorice Root
Garlic
Bee Propolis

The brand, "Now" makes a Propolis Plus Extract that contains, Licorice, Slippery Elm, Bee Propolis, Cloves, Goldenseal, Myrrh and Echinacea.

Long term use of Licorice Root may cause water retention, which will then cause high blood pressure.

GARLIC OIL TO RUB ON YOUR FEET

If you just don't like taking pills, tinctures, or drinking teas, good news. Rub it on your feet.

Several cloves of garlic

Olive oil

Mince garlic fine and let set for 10 minutes, Place in a jar and cover with olive oil. Let set 30- minutes to 12 hours. Rub the oil on the feet at night. Pull on an old pair of socks. Cover with another pair of socks.

Make fresh each day.

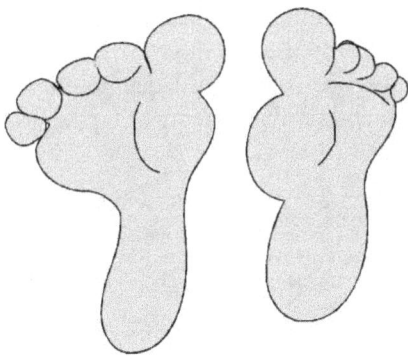

Garlic: When using garlic as an antibiotic or antimicrobial mince the garlic and let it set 10-15 minutes. The garlic cells must be ruptured to release two separate chemicals of the garlic, alliin and alliinase which then form a new compound called allicin.

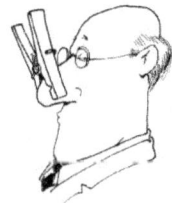

Yes you will smell like Garlic! Herbs that you put on your feet will go through your whole body and will come out your breath. You will reek of Garlic.
Maybe not an option when going to work.

FEVER

A fever is a beneficial immune system response. It is raising your normal body temperature of 98.6°f to over 99.9°f or more to kill and destroy the evil bacterial or virus invading your body.

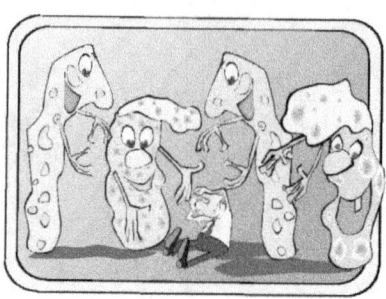

A low grade fever can be treated with herbs and fluids. Healthy adults do not need to take pills to stop the fever, but herbs to support the fever. Drinking hot teas and soups will help the diaphoretics (herbs that promote sweating) work better, and drinking plenty of liquids will prevent dehydration.

A fever will normally lasts 3-4 days. Seek medical help if fever lasts more than 3-4 days.

Consult your medical professional for high fevers. What is a high fever?

In healthy adults that is fever over 103-104° f.
Children under 3 months of age have a rectal temperature over 100.2°f.
Children 3-6 months have a rectal temperature over 101°f.
Children 4 months or older that have been immunized: a temperature over 102-103° f.

Bad Fever: seek medical help

If the person has serious health issues like cancer or HIV. The person stops taking fluids or shows signs of dehydration. The person becomes unresponsive. Fever over 103-104°f. Fever is accompanied by a stiff neck, is confused or having trouble staying awake. Severe pain in the lower abdomen, severe stomach pain, repeated vomiting, skin rashes, blisters, or a red streak in arm or leg, severe sore throat, swelling of the throat, persistent earache, pain with urination, back pain, shaking chills, severe cough, coughs up blood, has trouble breathing or seizures. When in doubt seek medical help.

People normally die from dehydration, not the fever itself.

Signs of dehydration:

Chapped lower lip when it wasn't there before is a sign of early dehydration. Clear or light colored urine means you are well hydrated, dark yellow or amber color urine is a usual sign of dehydration.
Push teas, broths, electrolyte replacement drinks, popsicles, etc

Other signs of dehydration:
Dry sticky mouth
Sleepiness or tiredness, children are likely to be less active than usual
Thirst
Decreased urine output
No wet diapers for three hours for infants
Few or no tears when crying
Dry skin
Headache
Constipation
Dizziness or lightheadedness

Severe dehydration: Seek medical attention

Extreme thirst
Extreme fussiness or sleepiness in infants and children
Irritability and confusion in adults
Very dry mouth, skin and mucous membranes
Little or no urination, urine that is darker than normal
Sunken eyes
The pinch test: Pinch the skin behind the wrist and pull up, it should return to normal when you let go. If it remains like a tent that is an indication of advanced dehydration, seek medical attention!
In infants, sunken fontanels – the soft spots on the top of the baby's head
Low blood pressure
Rapid heartbeat
Rapid breathing
No tears when crying
In serious cases: delirium or unconsciousness

If you do not have these conditions that require medical help, support your fever with hydration, plenty of fluids. Keep the feet warm and the head cool, not ice cold, just cool. A washcloth dipped in cool water or cool herbal tea placed on the forehead will work.

Use herbs depending on if it is hot external fever, or a cold external fever.

HOT EXTERNAL FEVER

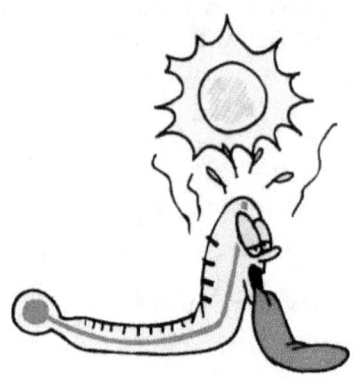

Feels hot inside and out
Might have a red tongue
Might have yellow phlegm coming up on the tongue
Might have a red sore throat
Might have a fast pulse

Treat with relaxing diaphoretics
A diaphoretics will dilate the capillaries to let the heat out. Diaphoretics will make you sweat.

Use teas and tinctures of these herbs either by themselves or any combination.
Chamomile
Elder flower, the flower not the berry
Yarrow
Lemon Balm
Lemon Grass
Hyssop
Peppermint especially effective for fever with nausea and vomiting
Boneset if you have intense aches and pains

Good Combination:
Elder flowers, Yarrow, Peppermint.
Boneset for pain
Tincture adult dosage: 2-4 ml (1/2-1 teaspoon) of the combination 3 times a day. Tea: Drink throughout the day.

COLD EXTERNAL FEVER

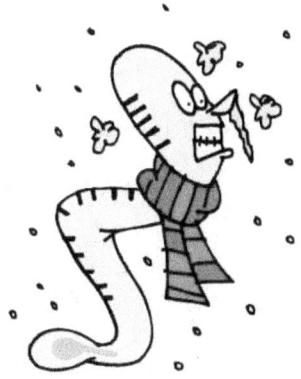

Cold to the bone
Shivering
Aversion to cold
Tongue is pale
White phlegm
Slow pulse
Itchy Throat

Do all you can to keep warm.
Bundle up.
Take a hot bath
Saunas are great.
Drink warm liquids with honey and lemon.

Use Stimulating diaphoretics. Stimulating herbs will warm you up from the inside out. Drink as teas all day long. If you prefer to take these as tinctures, drink some kind of hot liquid with the tinctures.

Ginger
Cayenne
Bee Balm
Yarrow
Peppermint
Boneset for pain
Tincture adult dosage: 2-4 ml (1/2-1 teaspoon) of the combination 3 times a day.

HOT, COLD, AND THEN HOT, COLD AGAIN

More likely than not you will be going back and forth between being hot or cold. Whichever symptoms you are effected by treat those symptoms.

Just Can't Take it Anymore?

Herbs to artificially lower the temperature and ease the pain.

Willow bark: anti-inflammatory
Meadowsweet flowers: aches and pain
Boneset, especially good for pain that goes all the way to the bone.

Willow bark and Meadowsweet flowers will lower your temperature and ease the pain. They contain salicylic acid, the chemical that has been synthesized by drug companies to produce aspirin.

Caution:
Children under 16 who have symptoms of flu or chicken pox
People with asthma, may stimulate bronchial spasms
People who are allergic to aspirin

Remember: this is not a religion. If this does not work for you, or do not have these remedies use the pharmaceutical remedies.

SEASONAL ALLERGIES

The number 1 herb for allergies is Ragweed, which is not easily found. The second choice, easily found herb for allergies is Nettles. Yes the stinging kind. Drinking it in a tea or taken as capsules will cause it to lose its sting.

Nettles is an excellent source of calcium and magnesium that is easily assimilated by your body, helping to build strong bones and teeth. Nettles is also a blood builder, a detoxing herb, good for the prostrate, helps prevent cramps by providing missing nutrients and helps with pain. Now what other allergy medicine can claim that?

Nettles is stimulating and a diuretic. Do not take close to bedtime.

Start taking nettles one month before you typically start getting the allergies or all year for the nutritional benefits.

If you are a tea drinker:
1 ounce of dried nettle
1 quart of boiled water
1 quart size container such as a mason jar
Place nettle in the container, pour the boiled water over the herb, cover and let set for 4-8 hours, or overnight.
Strain and drink throughout the day.
Optional: add peppermint or lemongrass or another herb of choice to improve the flavor

For those who are not tea drinkers, at least 2 capsules 2-3 times a day.

The freeze dried nettle leaf seems to work best for hay fever, 300 milligrams capsules 2-3 times a day.

Tinctures: 1-3 teaspoons daily

Nettles are a diuretic, so drink plenty of water.

Nettles are both drying and cooling.

If you have a dry constitution (dry hair, skin, always thirsty add a demulcent herb such as licorice root, slippery elm, plantain, marshmallow root).

If this herb makes you feel cold add ginger root.

Cautions: May interact with medication for high blood pressure, diabetes, anxiety or insomnia.

Anti inflammatory and Anti Allergy:
Licorice Root, not the DGL variety, acts much like cortisone.
Up to 6, 400-500 milligram capsules spread through the day.
Or 30-60 drops (1/4 to 1/2 teaspoon) of tincture up to 3 times per day.

Licorice Root contains a compound called glycrrhizin which can deplete the body's potassium levels, causing water retention, which can lead to high blood pressure.

Deglycrrhizinated Licorice Root (DGL) has been developed for those who need to take Licorice Root for extended periods of time.

Treat your symptoms the same as you do for colds and flu.

EAR ACHE

Ear Ache due to an infection use Mullein-Garlic oil available at most health food stores and online.

Warm oil to body temperature and then use a dropper to apply 3-4 drops into each ear. Place a cotton ball into each ear. Massage around the ear after applying the oil. Always treat both ears.

Use every 30 minutes or as needed. The excess oil will drain out of the ear.

Similasan ear drops. Available at most health food stores, drug stores, even Walmart.

Apply heat to the area. Wet a washcloth, heat in the microwave, place in a plastic bag, wrap in a dish towel and hold over painful ear. Or carefully use a heating pad.

Swimmer's Ear does not respond to oils.
Combine 1/4 cup of rubbing alcohol with several drops of Tea Tree or Lavender essential oils.
Shake well and use dropper to apply several drops into each ear. Massage the outside of the ear. Repeat several times a day.

Use Mullein/Lobelia Tincture make according to instructions for tinctures pg. 91 using 3 parts Mullein to 1 part Lobelia.

COLD SORES AND MOUTH SORES

Cold Sores:
Lemon Balm and Licorice Root,
Use these either as tinctures or Lip Balms

Mouth Sores: Low Alcohol Licorice Root Tincture
Apply to the sore or ulcer frequently, should heal the sore within 24 hours if applied early, may take 48 hours if you waited too long to apply.
The essential of Lemon Balm (Melissa) will work and be effective but is much too expensive to recommend.

Mouth Burns from hot food: Slippery Elm Powder mixed with honey.

Project: Lemon Balm Plus Salve, contains Lemon Balm, Calendula, St. John's Wort, and Licorice Root. Pg.117

Carolyn Gibson

3 First Aid

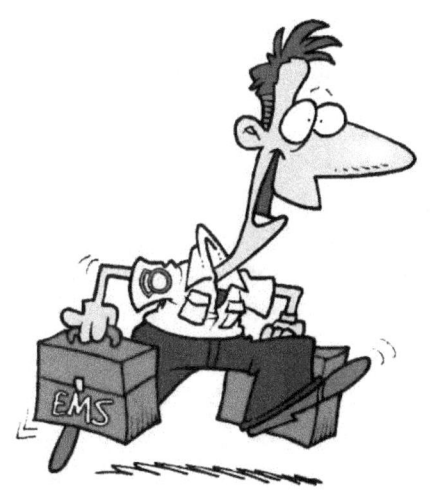

Insect, Stings and Bites: pg. 48
Burns and Sunburns: pg. 51
Booboos and Ouchies: pg. 53
Sprains, Strains and Bruises: pg. 55

INSECTS, STINGS AND BITES

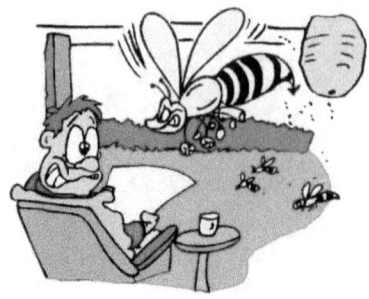

With insect bites and stings you are either trying to neutralize the venom in the sting, reduce the swelling or draw it out with poultices.

Ant Bites:
Rub in Vicks Vapor Rub or homemade version.
Or, apply essential oil of Peppermint to the area.

Mosquito Bite:
1 teaspoon of essential oil of Lavender mixed with 1 tablespoon of vegetable or nut oil.

Apply *Lemon Balm Plus Tincture pg. 102 or salve pg. 117*

Bees and Wasps and Scorpions:
Remove stinger from bee stings by scraping a credit card or other stiff object, (fingernails okay) across the sting. Using tweezers may press more venom into the skin. Bees are the only insects that will leave a stinger.

Rub area with ice cube for one minute. Wash with warm water.

Or, Prepared in Advance:
Washcloth
Water
5 drops of essential oil of Lavender
Dip a washcloth in water, wring out, dab the essential oil onto the washcloth. Store in a plastic bag in the freezer. Remove from the bag and apply on the sting area.

Or, apply honey to the sting site and leave on for 30 minutes and then rinse

OR, apply drops of Essential Oil of Peppermint to the area.
Herbal Remedies do not replace Benadryl for serious allergy reactions or an Epipen for anaphylactic episodes. Seek Medical Attention.

Onions
Slice an onion in half and lay on the sting area.
Or: Chop a fresh onion and lay on the area. Cover with gauze and tape on.

Bite and sting poultice
A poultice will pull out the poison out and keep it from spreading.
The Echinacea Root tincture will help reduce the allergic response and having a numbing effect, and the essential oils help reduce itching and swelling.

1 tablespoon of Echinacea Root Tincture pg. 99
1 tablespoon of distilled water or 1 tablespoon of Lemon Balm Tincture pg. 102
2-3 drops of essential oil of Lavender, Peppermint or Eucalyptus
1 tablespoon of Bentonite Clay or Green Clay
Combine water, tincture and essential oils. Slowly add to the clay stirring as the clay absorbs the liquid. This should make a paste tacky enough to stick to the skin. Store in a glass jar. If this should dry out add enough distilled water to reconstitute. Apply to sting area. Let dry for 30 minutes.

Quickly made: Clay poultice
Add 2 teaspoons of water to ½ teaspoon of clay

Itch Relief for Poison Ivy and Poison Oak, Chicken Pox

Clay poultice (prepare in advance and keep ready to use)
1 cup green volcanic clay or Bentonite Clay
Water or witch hazel
2 tablespoons of salt
3-5 drops of Essential oil of peppermint (enough to smell strong)

Mix the green clay and water or witch hazel to make a paste. Stir in the salt and essential oil of Peppermint. Store in a glass container. Apply to itching area, leave on for 30 minutes and then rinse with water or witch hazel. Reapply as needed.

Baking Soda Relief
1 teaspoon of baking soda
3 drops of essential oil of Lavender or Peppermint or Eucalyptus
Water
Put the baking soda in your hand, mix in the essential oils. Add enough water to form a paste that will stick to the skin. Spread on the itchy spot. Rinse after 30 minutes. Reapply as needed.

Spider Bites:

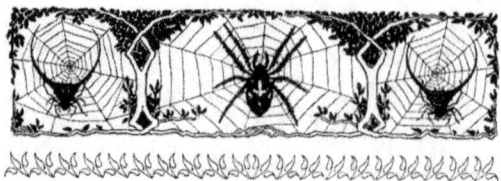

You normally do not know when a spider has bitten you. They have really small fangs and you cannot see the bite without a magnifying glass.

A brown recluse and hobo spiders cause local tissue damage. A brown recluse spider is tan or yellow brown, with a violin shaped mark on its back.

A black widow bite effects the nervous system. In normal cases the black widow's bite is too small to cause a problem. Symptoms that require medical attention are muscle spasms and cramps, nausea and vomiting and difficulty breathing. The black widow can be either black or brown and has a red hourglass shape on its underside.

You know you have been bit by a Brown Recluse or Hobo poisonous spider when the area starts swelling and you have an ulcer like wound that continues to grow and opening up. It could be a staph infection or it could be a spider bite. A Black Widow is different and this is **Not** a treatment for the Black Widow.

Apply an Activated Charcoal poultice and take a lot of ***Echinacea Root tincture***. Pg. 99.

ACTIVATED CHARCOAL POULTICE

A gauze bandage not the non stick
Activated Charcoal
Water
Self adherent stretchy tape
Optional: Sticky tape, paper or cloth
Bowl and stirring spoon or stick
A clean cloth to work on, charcoal is messy and will get all over everything.

Depending on the size of area, cut the gauze pad about the size of the area.

Add about 1-2 tablespoon of activated charcoal and add just a little water and stir. Keep adding water a little at time and stir. You want the consistency between a paste and a slurry. Spread the activated charcoal paste onto the gauze and apply to the injured area.

Wrap the self adherent tape around the gauze to keep in place. As an option you can then wrap the sticky tape around the self adherent tape to make sure it stays in place but do not place the tape on the skin. When you remove sticky tape, body hair will come out with the tape, leaving little holes for infection to re-enter the body.

Change the bandage once a day.

Echinacea Tincture pg. 99: 1-4 droppers full (1/4 to 1 teaspoon) every 2-4 hours the first day. The next half the dosage and the day after that half of that much.

If you are not getting better seek medical help.

BURNS AND SUNBURNS

Never put a salve, ointment or cream on a burn until the burn has first been cooled off. These things will hold the heat in.

First, cool the burn off by:
Soaking in cool water or
Using cold water compress,
A cool compress of diluted apple cider vinegar or
Spray with the Aloe Burn Spray

Aloe Burn Spray#1
Spray bottle
Equal amounts of Aloe Vera Juice and essential oil of Lavender
Mix together and keep in the refrigerator.
Pour over the burn or spritz it to cool it off. Shake well before using.
May be too strong for children and sensitive adults.

Aloe Burn Spray#2 less expensive
Spray bottle
4 oz. of Aloe Vera Juice
1/8 teaspoon of essential oil of Lavender
½ teaspoon of Vitamin E
Mix together and keep in the refrigerator.
Pour over burn or spray the burn to cool it off.
Shake well before using.

Honey Rescue
After skin is completely cool, cover with honey. Leave on for 30 minutes and reapply if necessary.
Optional: Add 2-3 drops of essential oil of Peppermint or Lavender to 1/4 cup of honey

Honey will seal off the air from the injury which will lessen the pain. Honey is antiseptic, and will help rehydrate the wound and prevent infection. Honey is antibacterial and healing.

Or apply the gel from a fresh **Aloe Vera Plant**

Or apply Wheat Germ oil or olive oil

Apply *All-purpose Healing Salve* pg. 118 or similar salves that contain St. John's Wort or Calendula flowers such as the Lemon Balm Plus pg. 117.

Burn on roof of mouth from hot food or drink
Mix Slippery Elm Powder with honey into a ball to suck on to heal the burn and lessen the pain.

Valerian, Willow, or Meadowsweet tincture taken internally to lessen pain.

Caution: Third degree burns require medical attention. If a burn shows signs of infection seek medical attention.

BOO-BOOS AND OUCHIES: MINOR CUTS AND SCRATCHES

Homemade remedy: All Purpose Healing Salve pg. 118

A little bleeding will help clean the wound. Apply a clean cloth with direct pressure to stop the bleeding. If not effective, use a Yarrow compress or Cayenne pepper directly on the wound.

After bleeding has stopped clean the area with soap and water, removing any debris that remains.
Soaking in hot water and soap would be the least painful.
Optional: Make a strong Yarrow tea to soak in

Clean with antiseptic solution:
Witch Hazel Extract with 6-8 drops of Tea Tree essential oil per 1 cup of extract, or

1 teaspoon tincture of Yarrow, mixed with 1/4 cup of water, Yarrow is also an anti inflammatory.

Hydrogen Peroxide mixed with equal amounts of distilled water.

Apply All Purpose Healing salve pg. 118

Cover with bandage to keep clean.
This is for minor injuries. Never use a salve for serious cuts.

Take tinctures of Valerian, Willow, or Meadowsweet if in pain.

Splinters:
Soak in Epsom salts to remove splinter or
Apply a thick clay poultice and change once or twice to remove splinter.

Disinfect with Witch Hazel Extract with Tea Tree essential oil.

Apply All Purpose Healing Salve pg. 118

Soothe your nerves with a tincture or tea of Valerian, Lemon Balm, or Chamomile.

Torn skin, skin folded back, abrasions:
After cleaning the wound, Use a Q-tip and salve or Vaseline to gently push the skin back into place. Use a waterproof transparent dressing to cover the area and protect from moisture and dirt.

Bee Propolis
Bee Propolis Tincture is sticky and makes a natural band aid that is also antiseptic. It will stick the skin together and form a natural waterproof barrier that will also let in oxygen.
This is a tincture made with alcohol, so it will sting.

You can also apply Propolis on top of your bandages to keep them from coming off due to moisture.

Rashes:
An ointment or salve made with Calendula flowers and Yarrow, Make an ointment using equal amounts of Calendula flowers and Yarrow. pg. 113

SPRAINS AND STRAINS AND BRUISES

The ultimate herbal remedy for strains, sprains and bruises are oils or salves made with either St. John's Wort or Arnica.
St. John's Wort and Arnica Oil should be available at your health food store. See recipes for making herbal oils pg. 110 and salves pg. 113

Bruise

A bruise is bleeding under unbroken skin. Some people bruise easier than others. Do not apply Arnica to broken skin.
Either St. John's Wort or Arnica Oil will work equally well.

OR
Soak a clean cloth in Witch Hazel and hold on the bruise for 15-20 minutes. Witch Hazel is an astringent. An astringent tightens the tissue which will reduce swelling and bleeding.

If the trauma causing the bruising seems serious seek medical attention.

Strains and Sprains:

A **sprain** involves the joints, this is when ligaments that hold the bones together that meet at the joint are pulled and overstretched. There is often bruising with a sprain.

A **strain** is when the muscle itself is pulled or overstretched. There can even be a little tear in the muscle.

Whichever one it is the treatment is the same.

The swelling or inflammation is the body's repair response. Inflammation creates swelling, redness, heat and pain. Increased blood rushes into the area creating redness and heat. Capillary walls let in more blood plasma and white blood cells which causes the swelling. The swelling puts more pressure on the nerves which causes the pain. The swelling and pain prevents you from moving the injured area. Pay attention to your body and do not use the injured area.

Visualize a cut in your hand where it bends at one of the fingers or thumb. If you keep that finger bent, the skin is staying together and healing. Every time you straighten that finger you are re-opening that cut. The same goes for a pulled muscle.
Stop using the injured area.

Apply ice packs to reduce the inflammation the first day or two, then switch to heat packs. If the injury is a hand or a foot soaking in cool water or cool herb tea will be most effective.

If you have a tincture of Arnica or St. John's Wort add it to the water. When using ice packs or cold water no more than 10 – 15 minutes at a time.

Elevated the injured area.

Apply either an Arnica or St. John's Wort salve, oil or liniment.

After the swelling has gone down alternating heat and cold will speed up the healing process.

Apply heat to the injured area for 15 minutes. This dilates the blood vessels bringing fresh new blood cells to nourish the area.

Then apply cold for 10 minutes. The cold constricts the blood vessels forcing out the old blood and toxins.

Then reapply the heat to bring in fresh new blood and then cold.

Repeat this process as often as you wish.

Apply Arnica or St. John's Wort salve or oil or liniment.

Make Oils pg. 110, Salve pg. 113, Liniments pg 106

Herbal remedies are a first response, not the only response. Always seek medical attention if there is a possibility of broken bones or if the sprain or strain is serious.

4 Pain

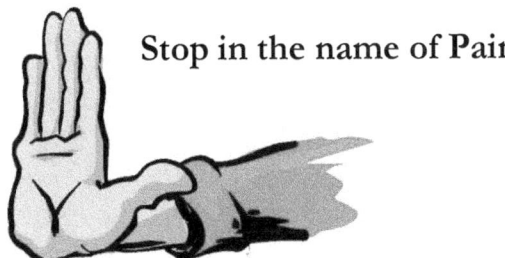 **Stop in the name of Pain**

Pain: the body is telling you that something is wrong. In some cases the body is telling you to stop what you are doing. Treating pain is not a matter of just a certain pill or tincture to stop the pain, but to address what is causing the pain.

Is it an obvious injury, is it chronic or did it come on out of the blue? Is the pain caused by infection, inflammation, or maybe tension and stress? Is it cramps? Treating tension and stress or cramps with anti-inflammatory will not give you relief. Treating an obvious injury with only an antispasmodic without the anti-inflammatory certainly will not work either. Herbal remedies are not always as effective as pharmaceutical drugs.

BACK SPASMS

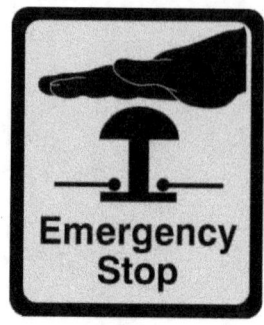

Maybe you just reached down to pick up a piece of paper and you get a grabbing sensation in your back that brings you to your knees. Did you overdue it the day before, or did you help move some furniture, or load firewood? Back spasms are normally caused by over doing an activity you normally do or doing an activity that you do not normally do.

Your back is saying stop!! But that does not mean complete bed rest after the first day.

Black Cohosh is the supreme herb for skeletal muscle spasms and is a natural muscle relaxer.

This is dose dependent. If using a tincture take a 1 ml (1/4 teaspoon). Wait another hour, if you do not get relief try another 1 ml (1/4 teaspoon) or even a teaspoon.

If using capsules try 3 capsules, wait an hour if you do not get relief try another 2 capsules. I personally take 5 capsules.

Black Cohosh can give some individuals frontal lobal headaches. If you have never taken Black Cohosh before take a few drops first to make sure it will not give you a headache.

Caution: Black Cohosh effects the hormones. Do not use if you are pregnant or nursing.

Other herbs that would help you relax would be Skullcap or Kava Kava.

Kava Kava not recommend if you are pregnant, nursing, liver disorder, or taking acetaminophen or prescriptions.

Exercise:

Complete bed rest will cause your muscle to stiffen up and prolong your recovery.

Not immediately, but maybe a few hours later or no later than the next day depending on how much pain you are in, start your exercise. Your muscles are either wanting you to compress the muscle or stretch the muscle.

Test which direction makes your back feel better.

If you cannot get out of bed, this may be as simple as bringing your knees to your chest. If that makes it worse, stop.

Try crossing one leg over your body, then the other. If either makes the pain worse than stop.

If you are able to roll over on your stomach do so and do a partial push up. Keeping everything from the waist down flat on the bed, push up with your arms.

If you can sit up in a chair, try bending over in the sitting position.
Does trying to touch your toes make it feel better, or bending backwards? Bending to one side or the other?
Whichever direction makes your back feel better do gentle stretching in that direction. Do not force the stretch. Just gentle stretches in that direction and you will find each time you can go a little further.

OTHER MUSCLE SPASMS

Maybe it is in the buttocks or the legs. Maybe it is not enough to bring you to your knees but it is uncomfortable and it hurts.

Black Cohosh is for all muscles.
Caution: not for pregnant women, has hormonal effects.
St. John's Wort Oil with essential oil of Lavender or Wintergreen applied externally to the muscle. Do not take internally.

Cramp Rub
2 oz. of St. John's Wort Oil or tincture
Add 8 drops of each essential oil of Lavender, Marjoram and Chamomile
Rub on the muscle as needed. Do not take internally.

Menstrual Cramps:

Lobelia tincture: 1 ml (1/4 teaspoon) at the first sign of cramps. Wait 10 minutes. If you still have the cramps take another 1 ml (1/4 teaspoon). Wait another 10 minutes. Another 1 ml (1/4 teaspoon) if needed. No more than 3 doses.

Follow with a cup of Peppermint tea or Cayenne capsules if it makes you too relaxed. If you are a coffee drinker, have a cup of coffee, or a tea drinker have a cup of hot or iced tea. Coffee and tea are herbs.

Lobelia is called the puke weed, because if you take too much it may cause nausea and vomiting.

Do not use if you are pregnant or nursing.

Leg Cramps

Herbs are not always the answer to leg cramps.

If you have done hard physical exercise or activity and have been sweating your cramps may be caused from dehydration or lack of potassium. Taking Black Cohosh will **not** help this kind of cramp when you obviously need water, salt or potassium.

Sometimes just a pinch of salt is all that you need.

Lack of water will make your muscles draw up.

Cramps may also be caused by not enough magnesium. Calcium makes your muscles contract, while magnesium make your muscles relax.

BACK ACHE

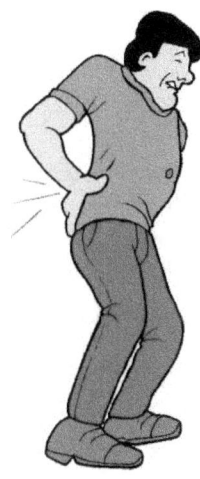

This could be due to tension, overuse, bad position of the body, bad bed, etc. it is an ache, it is uncomfortable but you can still function.

Back Ache due to Tension and Stress
Kava Kava, Passionflower, Valerian, Skullcap, or California Poppy, Lemon Balm: Dosage will vary. A little will help with tension maybe 1 ml (1/4 teaspoon) a lot may make you sleepy 5 ml (1 teaspoon). Try a 1 ml (1/4 teaspoon), wait an hour and take more if needed. Valerian:1/2 to 1 teaspoon maybe needed. Caution: Do not take Kava Kava, or Passionflower if pregnant or nursing. Do not take Kava Kava if you have a liver disorder, take prescriptions or acetaminophen. Passionflower may interfere with blood thinning medication.

Black Cohosh as a muscle relaxer may work. Do not use if pregnant or nursing.

St. John's Wort Oil with essential oil of Wintergreen applied to the spine on the low back. Do not take internally.

Hot bath with 1-2 cups of Epsom salts or 1 cup of apple cider vinegar. Optional: essential oils such as Lavender

Laying on a heating pad

General Back Ache:
Willow Bark or Devil's Claw
Caution: using Willow Bark
Children under 16 who have symptoms of flu or chicken pox
People with asthma, may stimulate bronchial spasms
People who are allergic to aspirin

SCIATICA NERVE PAIN

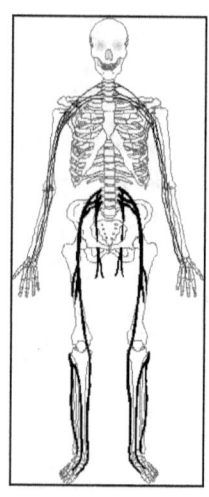

The sciatic nerve starts at L-4, (the low back) goes through the sacrum (the tail bone) continues through the muscles in the buttocks, runs alongside the hip joints, then goes on down through the thigh splitting at the knee all the way to the toes.

Sciatic nerve pain, is the pain in the buttocks, or in your hip, or hip joint. It can go down either side of your leg or behind your leg. This is the pain that keeps you tossing and turning all night long trying to get comfortable. This is the pain that makes a car ride or plain trip torture.

It can be brought on by prolonged sitting, or sitting without lumbar support, bending over or lifting heavy objects. It may be brought on by the slightest difference in shoe heel height or worn out heels, any circumstances causing you to tense up your buttock or leg muscles. Heavy lifting compressing your vertebrae or unresolved emotional issues may be causing this pain.

Sciatic nerve pain can be caused from tensed muscles in the buttocks squeezing the sciatic nerve, or compression of the lumbar disc or in my experience a combination of both.

Take St. John's Wort for the nerve that is being irritated and inflamed. Apply: St. John's Wort Oil with a few drops of the essential oil of Wintergreen applied to the spine on the low back.

If you have chronic sciatica pain take 1 ml (1/4 teaspoon) of St. John's Wort tincture internally 3 times a day.

Try Black Cohosh to relax the muscles in the buttocks and legs.

If you are hurting and you are agitated and stressed out, add one of the relaxing herbs, Kava Kava, Valerian , Lemon Balm or California poppy. Caution: Do not take Kava Kava, or Passionflower if pregnant or nursing. Do not take Kava Kava if you have a liver disorder, take prescriptions or acetaminophen. Passionflower may interfere with blood thinning medication.

Try the Mckenzie Push Up, illustrated on my website: www.FamilyGuidetoHerbs.com link to Self Massage Body Treatments.

Trigger Point you can do yourself with body tools or self massagers are in my book, Trigger Point Made Easy.
Available on my website or on Amazon.com.

Knee pain
Applying St. John's Wort Oil or Tincture with the essential oil of Wintergreen can also be effective for knee pain. If you also have pain in the front of the legs this could also be originating from the knee and this would be effective. Never take essential oil of Wintergreen internally.

Willow Bark Tincture or Elixar: 1 teaspoon every 2 hours, or Meadowsweet Tincture or Elixar, 30-60 drops (1/4 to1/2 teaspoon) as needed.

Caution:
Children under 16 who have symptoms of flu or chicken pox
People with asthma, may stimulate bronchial spasms
People who are allergic to aspirin

If these are not working, you may need to take a pharmaceutical solution like Advil or Aleve for the inflammation or even a prescription anti-inflammatory. You may need a prescription muscle relaxer for a brief period of time.
The danger to the body is taking these drugs daily.

This is not a religion. Do not suffer needlessly trying to prove that herbs work.

CHRONIC PAIN

Chronic pain due to arthritis or other inflammation:
Remember the meaning of any word that has "itis" in it means inflammation. If you do not have inflammation, your pain could be tension and not arthritis. Try the herbs recommended for stress and tension, Kava Kava, Valerian, California poppy and Skullcap. See precautions previous page.

Turmeric is an excellent herb for inflammation. It not only reduces inflammation but also helps reduce pain by depleting the substance P in the nerve endings. Substance P communicates pain to the brain.

Turmeric is taken internally but can also be used externally. Although effective externally it will stain the skin yellow. It can also be most effective by just using it in your diet every day.

Turmeric is drying to the body. If you have a dry constitution (dry skin, dry hair, feel thirsty, add a demulcent herb such as licorice root, marshmallow root, slippery elm, plantain honey and nut butters).

Enjoy Turmeric in your diet with 1-30 grams of Turmeric powder a day. Start off slow. Too much at once can make you nausea and give you indigestion.

Standardized extracts: 1-2 grams per day in divided doses.

Caution: Turmeric thins the blood so use caution if you are on blood thinners, have blood clotting issues, known gallstones, pregnant or nursing.

5*Loxin in Osteo Bio-Flex Joint Shield is Bosweilla, otherwise known as Frankincense.

Hops known as the sleeping herb is also an anti-inflammatory. Purluxan makes a form of Hops that will not make you sleepy.
Caution: Hops has estrogen like chemicals, if you have had estrogen driven breast cancer or if it is in your family avoid hops.

HEADACHES

Vascular: caused by dilation of the blood vessels brought on by too much of the wrong food such as too many sweets, too much cold food, or alcohol.
Alkalize the body with salty foods.
A vascular headache should respond to salty foods within 15-20 minutes.

Tension: caused by stress and tension, dehydration, too much salt, low blood sugar, staying in a bad position for too long, excessive mental concentration.
Change your activity.
Drink fluids if you are dehydrated

Valerian tincture 1/4 teaspoon every half hour until the headache is gone.

Essential Oil of Lavender or Peppermint applied to the temple, forehead and behind the ears.
Caution: Be extra careful not to get around the eyes. Do not rub your eyes after applying the essential oils with your fingers. Water does not wash off essential oils. Use either alcohol or dilute with lotion.

Chronic Tension Headaches:
Trigger Point Therapy either done by a massage therapists or go to my website, www.FamilyGuidetoHerbs.com, or Amazon.com for my book, Trigger Point Made Easy. This book teaches you to apply Trigger Point Therapy to yourself using body tools or self massagers.

General Headaches:
Essential Oil of Lavender applied to the temple, forehead and behind the ears. Sprinkle a few drops of the essential oil of Lavender in cool water. Dip a cloth into the water, wring out and apply to forehead while laying down.
Essential oil of Peppermint or Eucalyptus applied to the temple, forehead and behind the ears. If you have sensitive skin dilute in vegetable or nut oil before applying, 12 drops in 1 ounce of oil.

Willow Bark or Meadowsweet tincture or elixir would work like an aspirin. If aspirins work for you try these.
Caution:
Children under 16 who have symptoms of flu or chicken pox
People with asthma, may stimulate bronchial spasms
People who are allergic to aspirin

EAR ACHE

Ear Ache due to an infection use Mullein-Garlic oil available at most health food stores and online.

Warm oil to body temperature and then use a dropper to apply 3-4 drops into each ear. Place a cotton ball into each ear. Massage around the ear after applying the oil.

Use every 30 minutes or as needed.

Similasan ear drops available at most health food stores, drug stores and even Wal-Mart.

Apply heat to the area. This can be a warm cloth, a heating pad, etc. Wet a cloth, heat in the microwave, and place in a plastic bag and then wrap in a dishcloth. Apply to painful ear.

Swimmer's Ear does not respond to oil.
Combine 1/4 cup of rubbing alcohol with several drops of Tea Tree or Lavender essential oils.

Mullein/Lobelia Tincture, Prepare following direction for making tinctures, pg. 91 using 3 parts Mullein and 1 part Lobelia.

Shake well and use dropper to apply several drops into each ear. Massage the outside of the ear. Repeat several times a day.

5 Sleep and Stress

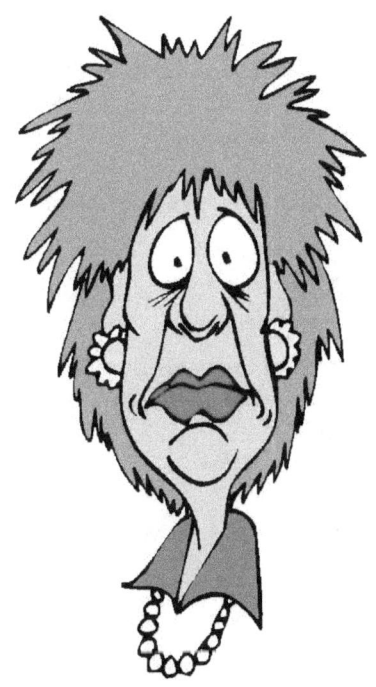

STRESS

Stress leads to high blood pressure, heart palpitations, inflammation, and cancer, loss of sleep, digestive problems and tension which leads to pain.

Even though stress causes all of these dangerous side effects it is a necessary part of living.

Stress creates strong bones, hardens our muscles, and fires up our immune system. Stress motivates us to go beyond our circumstances and make needed changes in our lives.

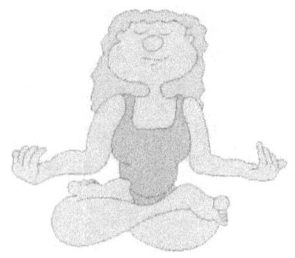

While meditation, a change of attitude, prayer, and deep breathing, is definitely effective, it is easier said than done.

These take time, practice and persistence.

As Christians, we firmly believe "that all things work together for good for those that serve the Lord", and we have complete peace that all things are in his hands, we still experience stress.

And we know:
"Cast your cares upon Jesus because he cares for you." I Peter 5:7

Matthew 6: 25-34 has a whole passage about worry.

And,

"do not be anxious about anything, but in everything, by prayer and petition, with thanksgiving, present your requests to God. And the peace of God which transcends all understanding, will guard your hearts and minds in Christ Jesus." Philippians 4:6-7

We may have complete peace and faith knowing "I can do all things through Christ who strengthens me."

"But!"

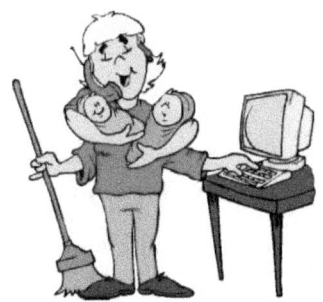

Trying to accomplish the many things we need to do stresses us out to the max.

The fact is, dealing with other people, families, friends, co-workers, automated phone systems, we get stressed out.

We may need to learn to say "no".

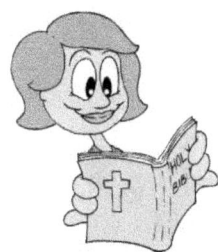

As we continue to pray, study His Word, grow in our Christian walk and rely on the Lord; we use the many plants God has given to deal with stress and anxiety.

While chemical drugs deaden the nervous systems, herbs nourish and support the nervous system.

Herbs may not work as quickly as the chemical drugs, they will be safer, have less side effects and with consistency and a good diet, resolve the issue.

Dealing with stress is more than just taking a potion or pill to relieve stress. Diet is important, herbs do help to nourish the nervous system but your body may need other nutrients. B vitamins and calcium are important nutrients for the nervous system.

B vitamins are in whole grains, egg yolks, leafy greens, beans, meat and seafood and dairy products. Oatmeal is great for the nerves.

Calcium is essential for our nervous system preventing nervousness, irritability, muscle spasms, muscle cramps and insomnia. Calcium is in dairy products, leafy greens, seaweed and many herbs.

All the feel good foods that we crave, sugar, caffeine, alcohol and processed foods deplete the nervous system.

Exercise, God made our bodies to move. Exercise provides essential oxygen and circulation.

If you are not getting enough sleep you will be stressed and if you are stressed you cannot sleep. The same herbs that are for stress and also for sleep, the dosage would be increased for sleep.

Herbal remedies for stress can be divided into two categories. If this a long term or chronic stress situation you made need to take nervine herbs as a daily tonic. If this is more less as something that pops up occasionally and you need a quick fix.

All herbs work for some people and no herbs work for all people. You will have to discover through experience which of the many herbs work for you.

Dosages can be tricky. Some people are very sensitive to any herbs for stress and need very little while others require quite a bit. Start with the least amount and add more if needed.

Daytime agitation: When you get to going too fast and just can't slow down or get tightness in your chest or slight pain in the chest.

The mildest and most recommended for those that are sensitive, children and elderly would be, California Poppy and German Chamomile and the essential oil of Lavender. Stronger herbs would be Valerian, Lobelia, Lemon Balm, and Passionflower.

German Chamomile is the most used herbal tea in the western world.
When using the tea medically let steep for 10 minutes.
German Chamomile Tincture
1-4 ml (1/4 teaspoon - 1 teaspoon) 3 times a day.

California Poppy Tincture:
.05 – 1 ml (8-30 drops) 3 times a day. 1-4 ml at night.

Essential Oil of Lavender: Some people can just smell Lavender and it will calm them instantly. I am not one of those person, you may be.

Valerian: safe, non-toxic, non-addictive.
Valerian may have the opposite effect on 5% of the population and make then hyper instead of relaxed. If Valerian has this effect on you discontinue use. If you have never tried Valerian try a few drops first to make sure it does not agitate you first.
1/2 to 1 teaspoon 1-3 times a day. Up to 2 teaspoons may be needed.
Can be combined with St. John's Wort for anxiety.

Lobelia: This is a low dose herb. 4-6 drops first. Wait 30 minutes.
Once you are accustomed to how much you can take, and depending on the quality and the strength of the Lobelia, you may need up to 1/4-1/2 teaspoon.

Lobelia is called the puke weed. Too much will cause nausea and vomiting.
Caution: Do not take if you are pregnant or nursing.
Follow with a cup of peppermint tea, or coffee if it makes you too relaxed.

Lemon Balm:
Especially good for heart palpitations due to anxiety.
As a therapeutic tea let it steep for 10-15 minutes and drink morning and night or as needed.
Tinctures: 2-6 ml (1/2 teaspoon – 1 ½ teaspoon) as needed.

Passionflower: do not take if pregnant, may interfere with blood thinning medications.
Especially good for nervous exhaustion.
1-4 ml (1/8 – 1 teaspoon) twice a day or 1-4 ml at night for sleep.

There are many formulas combining these herbs together creating a synergy between them making them more effective.

Insomnia:
There are countless formulas, below are some examples. You can certainly use your intuition to formulate and customize your remedy.
The below tea formulas can easily be made into tincture formulas, pg. 91, using glycerin for children's formulas pg. 104.

Children's Sedative Tea from Germany
30% Lemon Balm
30% Lavender flower
30% Passionflower
10% St. John's Wort

Adult's Sedative Tea from the Commission E
40% Valerian Root
30% Lemon Balm
30% Passionflower

Surprisingly, if you have trouble sleeping you don't just take the herbs before bedtime. Sometimes you need to take ½ teaspoon of the herb remedy 3 times a day, and then take a teaspoon at night.
If you wake up at 3 or 4 in the morning have a bottle with a dropper handy that you can easily roll over and take a dropper full or 2 and fall back to sleep.

It is all about doing what works for you.

When these do not work:
Try 1/2 teaspoon of St. John's Wort tincture 3 times during the day. 3 hours before bedtime start taking a combination of 1 teaspoon of Valerian and Hops tincture each hour until bedtime. (1/2 teaspoon of Valerian and 1/2 teaspoon of Hops) Hops is also an anti-inflammatory which will help if your insomnia is due to pain. **Caution: Do not use Hops if you have a family history of breast cancer. Safety in pregnancy unknown.**

Essential Oil of Lavender

Apply a few drops of Lavender on the bottom of your feet or pillowcase.

Make a Lavender spray with 10 drops of essential oil of Lavender, 7 tablespoons of water and optional 1 tablespoon of Vodka as a preservative and spray the bed sheets at night.

Add the essential oil of Lavender to a hot bath at night.

Sleep Pillow

An old fold remedy going back to King George, Abraham Lincoln and the Prince of Wales is a sleep pillow. This is not a full size pillow but a small pillow you place inside the pillowcase.

Make a small pillow and stuff with Hop Strobiles, Lavender flowers and optional Rose petals. Adding Mugwort to the blend is said to cause vivid dreams.

For this to work you smell the Lavender and the Hops. The only way to release the scent is to punch or squeeze the pillow. So when you wake up during the night you need to punch or squeeze the pillow.

Children:

Make a small doll or pillow and stuff with Hops, Lavender and Dill seed.

6 Tummy Alert

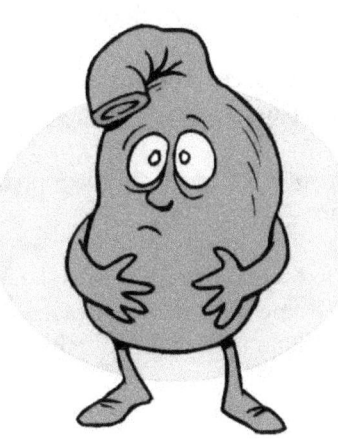

Constipation pg. 74

**Nausea & Vomiting,
Gas & Bloating pg. 75**

Diarrhea pg. 76

This will not cover chronic problems like inflammatory disease, Crohn's disease, irritable bowel syndrome, etc. but the digestive problems that pop up now and then.

CONSTIPATION: DIFFICULTY PASSING STOOLS.

Lack of fiber is not the only cause of constipation but is the most common. Insufficient water and not enough good fats in the diet can also be a cause.

Add more greens to your diet. If you do not like greens try the green powder capsules or adding green powders to your smoothies.

Too many carbohydrates. Notice after celebrating a holiday besides having a sugar hangover you are also constipated?

Stress can cause constipation, as can certain medications and mineral supplements, nerve damage, hypothyroidism and even antihistamines.

Lack of exercise. Your body was designed to move. The intestines require movement to function correctly. Sometimes just walking will help.

When adding more fiber to your diet bring plenty of water. Not enough water with your fiber will cause constipation.

Psyllium seed husk (the active ingredient in Metamucil) is the most common form of bulk forming laxatives. Remember plenty of water. Drinking with apple juice will make the Psyllium seed more effective.

If you are pass that point and need immediate relief:
Senna, is the most used laxative in the world. After that is Cascara Sagrada. These are stimulants and should only be used as a last resort and not on a regular basis.

The safest ways to take these harsh laxatives is combined with gentler herbs like fennel seed and licorice root. Take these according to package directions.

NAUSEA AND VOMITING, GAS AND BLOATING

These are lumped together because you will use the same carminative herbs. They relieve gas by helping to dispel the gas, calm the intestines and are antispasmodic.

Ginger
Ginger tea, Crystallized Ginger Candy, a good Ginger Ale will help. *Ginger Oxymel pg.121*

Ginger is the number one choice for motion sickness and is as effective as Dramamine and will not make you sleepy.
For motion sickness take capsules equal to 1500 milligrams 30 minutes before travel.
Caution: Pregnant women should not take more than 1 gram of powdered Ginger per day. Use caution if you are on blood thinners. May cause heartburn.

If you cannot handle Ginger, try **Peppermint** tea, only steep for 2 minutes. Try Peppermint lozenges or candy.
Avoid taking Peppermint internally if you have esophageal reflux or heartburn. Try Peppermint externally.

Essential oil of **Peppermint** or **Patchouli** diluted 50/50 with carrier oil, massage behind the ears and around the navel 2-3 times daily.
A drop or 2 of essential oil of Peppermint on the lips or tongue.

Other herbs to consider or add to the mixture are Fennel seeds, Dills seeds, Caraway seeds.

Licorice Root Tincture: Licorice Root is a mild laxative, sometimes moving the bowels slightly will help move the gas on out.

Lobelia Tincture
2-3 drops will calm the stomach and stop dry heaves. 2-6 drops to stop vomiting. Depending on the formula up to ¼ teaspoon may be needed.
Caution: Too much will cause vomiting, do not use if pregnant

Project: Slippery Elm Throat and Tummy Soothers pg. 122. Or Ginger Throat and Tummy Soother pg. 127 or Peppermint Patty Throat and Tummy Soother, pg. 128
Caution: Do not give or apply Peppermint to children under 3.

Vomiting

Activated Charcoal:
1-2 large spoonfuls of charcoal mixed with a small amount of water. If you can follow with a glass of water. If you throw this up, take it again. Take up to 3 times.

If you are taking the activated charcoal for gas, save this for extreme times when the other remedies have failed.

Seek medical attention if:
Vomit contains bright red blood.
Vomiting follows an injury to the abdomen.
Vomiting accompanied with abdominal pain or the abdomen is tender to the touch.
Vomits more than once after a head injury.
Vomiting is persistent especially in infant or small child.
Vomit accompanied by signs of dehydration:
Dry mouth, sunken eyes, severe thirst, decrease in amount of urine, irritability. The pinch test pg. 39
Child recovering from the flu or chicken pox and has persistent vomiting along with behavioral changes.
Vomiting has not stopped within 12 hours.
Develop a fever higher than 103°f.
Vomiting with Diarrhea: Seek medical attention

Diarrhea without vomiting and Person is not diabetic.
Diarrhea: urgent, frequent, watery bowel movements, the body is trying to get rid of something. Day one, let the body do its job. If your diarrhea has not responded to herbal treatment after 2 days seek medical attention.

All diarrhea causes you to lose water and minerals. If you do not replace the water and the lost minerals you will become dehydrated and have an electrolyte imbalance which can lead to nervous system disorders.

People all over the world die of dehydration not the diarrhea itself. You need, water, sugar (refined sugar, not honey or molasses), and salt.

Rehydration Formula: 1 quart of water, 6 teaspoons of refined sugar, 1/2 teaspoon of salt.

Or: Emergence C or sports drink

Cramps and spasms with diarrhea: Caution if pregnant or breast feeding. Wild Yam tincture, this is not sweet potatoes or yams from the grocery store. 1/2 dropper full until the cramps stop. If this is not working try an anti spasmodic like Valerian.

Stopping diarrhea:

Strongest remedy: Blackberry root bark tincture

½ teaspoon ever 30 minutes. Even though Blackberry root tincture is on the FDA's safety list you may not find this in the stores.

2nd on the list: Blackberry, Blueberry or Raspberries or Bilberries jellies, wines, or jams if the seeds have been removed (seeds will have a laxative effect).

These berries have tannins which tighten and tone the intestinal lining, which prevent the toxic or irritating substances from being reabsorbed into the intestines.

Take a 2 spoonfuls every 30 minutes until the diarrhea stops.

Berry remedy for diarrhea:

3 heaping tablespoons of dried berries
2 cups of water
Bring water and berries to a boil and simmer for 15 minutes. When the mixture has cooled, strain and bottle and store in the refrigerator. Take 2 tablespoons ever 30 minutes until diarrhea stops.

Yarrow tincture: 10-15 drops 3 times a day.

Mild Diarrhea: Meadowsweet

Causes:

Chronic conditions: like inflammatory bowel diseases and irritable bowel diseases. These conditions require a skilled medical professional for the root cause, you can treat the symptoms.

Try activated charcoal. 4-6 capsules between meals 3 times a day.

Herbs that are nerviness or anti-spasmodic:

Best for the gut: Chamomile, Catnip, Meadowsweet, use individually or combined.

Teas are best, alcohol or glycerin tinctures will work.

Infectious: bacteria, bad food or water

You are not trying to stop the diarrhea because the body needs to get rid of the bacteria...

Activated charcoal will absorb the pathogens and the toxins that they create.

Activated charcoal will also absorb any herbs or medications also. So wait at least 20 minutes after giving herbs or medications before giving the charcoal.

Activated charcoal for diarrhea:
1-2 teaspoons of activated charcoal per ½ cup of water, should be a thin slurry
Drink this 2-3 times the first day.
Or: Activated charcoal capsules:
2 capsules 3 times a day.

Non infectious: stress, food allergies, medication
Stress related diarrhea: Use herbs that are calming: nervines or anti-spasmodic.
Best for the gut: Chamomile, Catnip, Lemon Balm, or Meadowsweet, use individually or combined. Valerian, and Lobelia can work.
Teas are best, alcohol or glycerin tinctures will work.

Seek Medical attention if:

Diarrhea last more than 3 days.
Babies younger than 6 months, more than a day.
Signs of dehydration:
Dry mouth, sunken eyes, severe thirst, decrease in amount of urine, irritability. Pinch test, pg. 39
Severe abdominal pain
Fever over 101°f
Prolonged diarrhea after a camping trip or traveling overseas.

Activated Charcoal:
If you do not drink enough water with charcoal or just have a sensitive digestive system it can be constipating.
Drink more water and cut your dosage in half.

7 Women's Concerns

Not to be confused with women complaining.

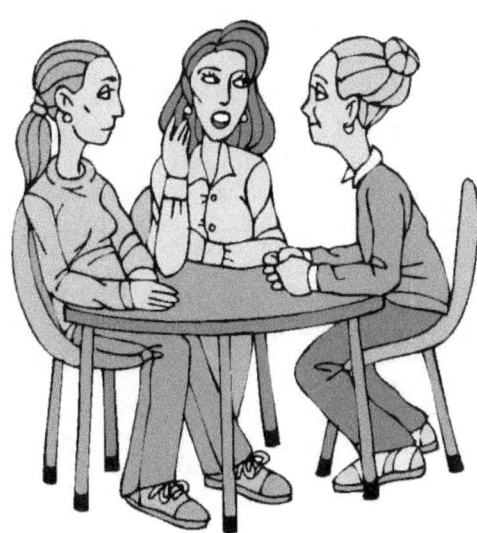

BREAST TENDERNESS

Mullein and Lobelia:
3 parts Mullein to 1 part Lobelia
Tincture, salve or oil applied to the breast each night along with taking a tincture 3 times a day
Prepare oil pg. 110 or salve according to directions on pg.113, 3 parts Mullein and 1 part Lobelia
Prepare tincture according to directions on pg. 91 using 3 parts Mullein and 1 part Lobelia. Or make a tea.

Hot and Cold Compresses:
Apply a hot compress for 5 minutes and then a cold compress for 5 minutes. Alternate for 30 minutes

MENSTRUAL PAIN

There are many herbs and combination of herbs to try to see which one will work for you. Caution: Do not use these if you are pregnant without medical supervision..
Cramp bark, Black Haw, and Valerian Combination
4-8 ml (1/2 – 2 teaspoons) of tincture 3 times a day

Cramp bark with Yarrow
½ teaspoon – 1 teaspoon every hour until cramps are relieved

Cramp Rub
2 oz. of St. John's Wort Oil or tincture
Add 8 drops of each essential oil of Lavender, Marjoram and Chamomile
Rub on abdomen as needed.

Lobelia tincture: 1 ml (1/4 teaspoon) at the first sign of cramps. Wait 10 minutes. If you still have the cramps take another 1 ml (1/4 teaspoon). Wait another 10 minutes. Another 1 ml (1/4 teaspoon) if needed. No more than 3 doses.

Follow with a cup of Peppermint tea or Cayenne capsules if it makes you too relaxed. Coffee or tea would be fine.

Lobelia is called the puke weed, because if you take too much it may cause nausea and vomiting. Do not use if you are pregnant or nursing.

VAGINAL AND VULVA IRRITATION

When treating "down under" you can't see the problem so you have to feel the problem.

Balms and salves made with Lemon Balm and Licorice Root will help relieve symptoms of the occasional irritation of the vaginal or vulva area.

Non alcohol based tinctures of Lemon Balm (Melissa) and Licorice Root is helpful. Remember where you are putting it. Alcohol would burn. If an alcohol tincture of Lemon Balm or Licorice Root is all that you have, mix it with lotion or salve to reduce the sting of the alcohol.

A strong Lemon Balm tea in a cool sitz bath would be the most effective but takes a little more time.

Lemon Balm's anti-histamine properties make it especially good applied to soothe the itch. Nettles is also a natural antihistamine. Take 2 capsules up to 3 times a day. Nettles will also act as a diuretic, so I do not recommend taking it close to bedtime.

If these do not work try and over the counter antihistamine like Benadryl.

Lemon Balm's nervine properties makes it soothing to the vaginal area.

If we are stressed out, it will often show up in this sensitive area much like cold sores or fever blisters show up on the mouth.

Licorice Root tincture (a low alcohol preparation) is good if there is a blister, an ulcer, a sore or maybe an ingrown hair. Licorice Root is an anti-inflammatory and its mucilage properties (slippery) is healing to mucus membranes. Licorice Root tincture applied to the area will usually heal the area within 24 hours, or up to 48 hours if you waited too long to apply it.

Both Lemon Balm and Licorice Root have anti-viral properties that research has proven to be effective against the herpes virus and supports the immune system.

Project Remedy: Lemon Balm Plus Salve or the Oil (pg. 117) contains both Licorice Root and Lemon Balm. It also contains St. John's Wort for nerve pain. Does anyone doubt the abundance of nerves in this area? The Calendula in this formula is a gentle herb that acts as an antiseptic, assists in cell repair, and is specific for skin ulcers.

Remember: This is oil based with Beeswax. Wear a panty liner to protect your good underwear. Or apply dish washing liquid to the panty area prior to washing.

A strong tea of Echinacea Root in a cool sitz bath may have a numbing effect on the painful area.

Echinacea Root Tincture applied directly would burn this gentle area. The tincture could be put in hot water letting the alcohol evaporate, cool and then use in a sitz bath. Try an Echinacea Root infused oil.

There may be a time that a Mullein/Lobelia salve may work better. Prepare according to directions for making oils pg. 110 or salves pg. 113 using 3 parts Mullein and 1 part Lobelia.

Often times you will need to switch around for which remedy works best.

To make these remedies more effective put on a long dress or gown and go without underwear for a day or night.

Take 1/4 to ½ teaspoon of **Lemon Balm Plus Glycerite** pg. 105 throughout the day. This is a yummy tincture which could also be applied to the vulva area if you do not need an oil.

VAGINAL OR VULVA DRYNESS:

Almond oil is the choice for vaginal or vulva lubrication, especially for sex.

Lemon Balm Plus oil pg. 116 or salve will work great, pg. 117.

There are many women's herbs to combat vaginal dryness, which take up to 3 weeks to see if they are going to work. There are many herbal books written for menopause and vaginal dryness.

I personally take bio-identical hormones which are plant based and do require a prescription. I found my doctor by going to a compounding pharmacy and asking them which doctors used their services. This led to me being part of a 4 year research program verifying the safety and effectiveness of bio identical hormones.

Only a compounding pharmacy will fill a prescription for the bio identical hormones. The national chain based pharmacies will not fill the prescriptions for natural hormones.

8 Making Herbal Remedies

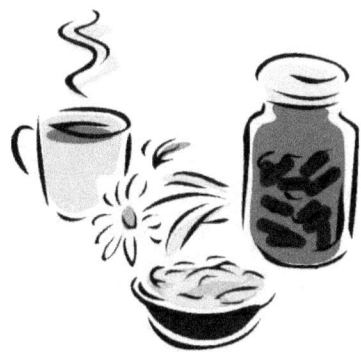

Choosing which method to extract the healing properties of any given herb will depend on if the "active ingredient" is water soluble or alcohol soluble. Water soluble herbs can be taken as a tea. If the "active ingredient" is alcohol soluble it will be more therapeutic taken as a tincture. There are herbs that can be effective that are soaked in oil or glycerin. Today's newest technology extracts herbs by carbon dioxide, called super critical CO_2 promises to be the most exact and best form of extraction, but is not a home project.

Pills and capsules are a choice. Simply rolling an herbal powder inside a ball of peanut butter or almond butter will work.

For many of us," are we a tea person?", or would we rather take a pill or tincture or extract.

In some instances we need a salve or an oil for external application. Sometimes we can just incorporate herbs into our diets.

Allopathic or chemical medicines normally have only one benefit. Herbs can have many different benefits and sometimes seem opposite to each other. Peppermint and Lavender can be both relaxing and stimulating. When you see a list of herbs to treat certain conditions, you must consider what is causing the symptoms. Herbal remedies are more effective in some forms than others.

When you inhale Peppermint it does help with sinus congestion. But you can smell it all day long and it is not going to help your pain except for certain headache-like-sinus congestion. But for most headaches and muscle pain, it has to be massaged into the muscle. In this case an essential oil of Peppermint would be more effective.
Drinking a cup of Peppermint tea, or sucking on a Peppermint candy would work better for an upset stomach.

Ginger is more effective taken internally for nausea that being rubbed on as an essential oil.

For me menstrual cramps or intestinal cramps are better relieved taking Black Cohosh or Lobelia internally than having an essential oil rubbed onto my belly.

When buying herbs, they are usually cut and sifted, powdered or whole. The whole herb would retain more of its properties and stay the freshest the longest. You would then need to chop or powder them before use.

Chopped and sifted are preferred for making teas and tinctures, and oils. Powdered herbs are for making herbal pills, lozenges, and capsules. They can be used for tinctures, teas and oils but are harder to strain.

DOSAGE

How much is a drop? How much is an ml?

½ ml = 8 drops = 1/8 dram
5/8 ml = 10 drops = 1/8 teaspoon = 1/6 dram
1 ml = 30 drops
1 1/4 ml = 20 drops = 1/4 teaspoon = 1/3 dram
2 ½ ml = 40 drops = ½ teaspoon =2/3 dram
5 ml = 150 drops = 1 teaspoon = 1/3 tablespoon = 1 1/3 dram
10 ml = 300 drops = 2 teaspoons =
15 ml = 1 tablespoon = 3 teaspoons = 4 drams
30 ml = 1 fluid ounce
500 ml = 500 grams = ½ kilo= 16 fluid ounces = 1 pint
1000 ml = 1 liter

1 tablespoon = 3 teaspoons
4 tablespoons = 1/4 cup= 2 fluid ounces
5 1/3 tablespoons = 1/3 cup
8 tablespoons = ½ cup = 4 fluid ounces
12 tablespoons = ¾ cup = 6 fluid ounces
16 tablespoons = 1 cup = 8 fluid ounces
1 fluid ounce = 2 tablespoons
1 cup = ½ pint = 8 fluid ounces
2 cups = 1 pint = 16 fluid ounces
4 cups = 2 pints = 1 quart =32 fluid ounces
4 quarts = 1 gallon = 128 fluid ounces

1/4 teaspoon = 1.25 ml
½ teaspoon = 2.5 ml
1 teaspoon = 5 ml
1 tablespoon = 15 ml
1/4 cup = 60 ml
1/3 cup = 80 ml
½ cup= 120 ml
1 cup = 235 ml

SUGGESTED CHILDREN DOSAGE

The herbal remedies in this book is written primarily for adults. I feel like most parents will need to first try these remedies on themselves and have complete confidence in these remedies before trying them on their children.

Below is a suggested conversion for children if the adult dosage is 1 teaspoon:

Younger than 3 months: 2 drops

3-6 months: 3 drops

6-9 months: 4 drops

9-12 months: 5 drops

12-18 months: 7 drops

18-24 months: 8 drops

2-3 years: 10 drops

3-4 years: 12 drops

4-6 years: 15 drops

6-9 years: 24 drops

9-12 years: 30 drops

TEAS

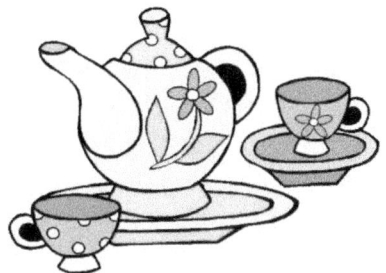

1 teaspoon of dried herb

Or 3 teaspoons of fresh herb

To 1 cup of water

For centuries herbs (fresh or dried) were drank as teas. This is the simplest method and sometimes the most effective. Teas are drunk all through the day and night. Typically 1 cup three times a day. These teas can be used as a compress, or as a poultice or poured into a bath. They can also be used as douches or enemas, make sure the tea is cooled to room temperature before use. They are made fresh each day as they will spoil.

Sometimes just the ritual of taking the time to stop and make a cup of tea or coffee would be part of the relaxing effect. Everyone knows that coffee is a stimulant, but how many people will relax with a cup of coffee?

Leaves, flowers, green stems, roots, bark and some seeds of the plants are used. If the herb is fresh it must be chopped in to tiny pieces. If the herb is dried it is crushed either with a mortar and pestle (old fashion method) or today's method would be a food or coffee grinder.

Hot Infusion

Infusions are used to extract the medical properties from leaves, flowers and soft stems. A glass or china teapot is first warmed with hot water, 1 teaspoon of dried herb or 3 teaspoons of fresh is added to the tea pot and 1 cup of boiling water is poured over the herb. The teapot is then covered with a lid and is allowed to steep for 10-15 minutes for the herb's medical properties. For taste only, steep for 3-5 minutes.

Cold Infusion

Cold infusions are used for herbs that are sensitive to heat and will lose their effectiveness. In this case, the herbs and water or milk are placed in a container with a tight fitting lid and allowed to sit for 4-12 hours. Do not use milk if the individual is allergic to milk.

Decoctions

When parts of the herb that is used is hard and woody such as the roots, rhizomes, bark, hard seeds, nuts, the mixture is brought to a boil and simmered for 10-15 minutes.

Of course there are always exceptions to the rules. Some roots contain volatile oils which would be destroyed by boiling. These herbs are finely chopped and infused with a tight fitting lid. Ginger, Saw Palmetto, and Turmeric come to mind.

If an herbal formula calls for both the leaves and flowers or a plant and the roots of another, how would you prepare it?

TINCTURES OR EXTRACTS

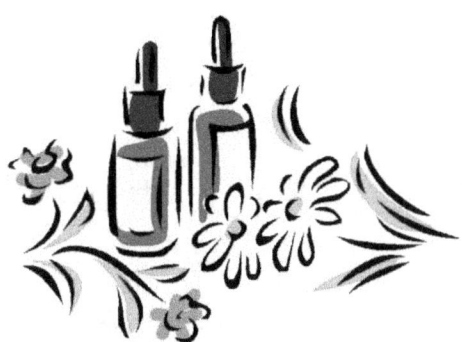

Alcohol or Vinegar Tincture

1 part Herbs
2 -3 parts Vodka or Everclear, or Apple Cider Vinegar
Shake daily for 2-6 weeks.
Strain

Tinctures are made with alcohol or vinegar. Sometimes they are mistakenly called extracts. Tinctures are more concentrated than teas, so use less, and the alcohol or the vinegar acts as a preservative. Tinctures stored in a cool dark place may have a shelf life up to 10 years.

Commercially made tinctures have an exact ratio of alcohol to herb varying with each herb and different standards.

The Folk method or homemade tinctures are made by chopping or grinding the herbs, filling any size jar half way with dried herbs and then filling the jar to the top with 60-80 proof Vodka or 190 Proof Vodka or Everclear Everclear is preferred when using bark, seeds and roots. Everclear can also be used when making tinctures with leaves and flowers, it is more expensive than using Vodka.

When using fresh herbs, allow the herbs to wilt all day or overnight to reduce their moisture content. Fill the container all the way and then mash them down about halfway.

If the herbs are powdered I will fill the container 1/4 of the way. If using a combination, I use my best guess.

Place a tight fitting lid on the jar and label with the name of the herb, the solvent used, and the date. Shake, and then check in a few hours to make sure the herbs are completely covered with the solvent adding more if necessary.

Place out of direct sunlight, and shake daily for 2-6 weeks.

Check this mixture the first few days to make sure the solvent completely covers the herbs, add more solvent if necessary. There should be enough solvent to shake the contents to mix. If the herbs are packed tight in the jar and you cannot shake to mix, add more solvent.

It is then strained and poured into dark colored bottle with a tight fitting lid and labeled.

Why 2-6 weeks? David Hoffman's protocol for making herbal medicine is 2 weeks. Rosemary Gladstar states 4-6 weeks. Many other herbalists recommend 6 weeks.

Since the strength of a homemade tincture will vary these are used when the dosage is not critical.

Tinctures can be taken straight, added to water or other liquids, used to make ointments, salves, suppositories and lozenges.

Important tinctures to have on hand would be Echinacea for wounds, infections, colds and the flu. A tincture of Elderberries would go along with Echinacea for colds and flu if the sugar or honey in the Elderberry syrups is not wanted.

A tincture of Hops would be valuable to have on hand for insomnia and inflammation.

A tincture of Sage mixes well with water as a mouthwash for dental problems and fresh breath.

SUGGESTED EQUIPMENT

Canning jars, or small jars with lids
Jar lifter (available in canning department of stores.)
Funnel
Dark bottles
Strainers: re- useable coffee filters, jelly bags, cheesecloth
Measuring cups and spoons
Clean towel or paper towels
Double boiler, find an inexpensive double boiler at Bed, Bath and Beyond

Your herbal remedies are only as good as your preparation of them. Even though "Cleanliness is next to Godliness" is not biblical, it is important for safety and preservation.

I use the wide mouth canning jars because it is easier to put your hands into them for cleaning.

I use the plastic white caps that are now available for the canning jars.

PREPARING FRESH HERBS

Place in a sink filled with cold water.

Slosh around in the sink and let set for a few minutes.

Sand, dirt and other debris should settle to the bottom of the sink.

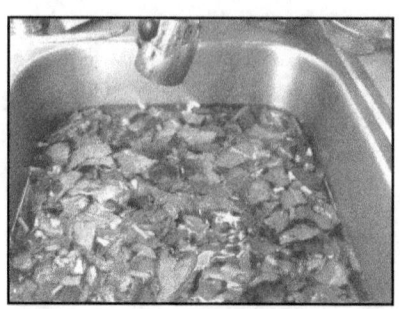

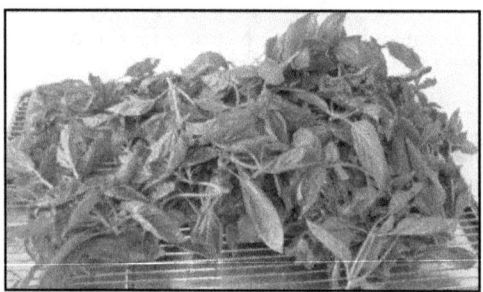

Lift herbs out of the sink and lay herbs out on a drying rack or towel to dry and wilt.

Too much moisture in your herbs will dilute the alcohol in your tincture.

I have a window air conditioner. I will often place the herbs in front of the air conditioner to hurry the drying process, turning the herbs several times.

Chop the herbs. The finer the herbs are chopped the more of the medical properties will be extracted.

PREPARING YOUR EQUIPMENT

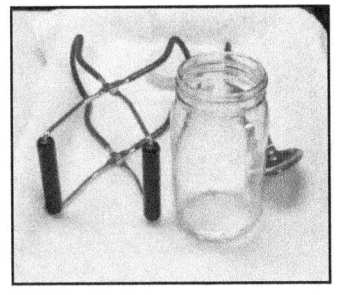

Lay out a clean towel to place your equipment on after you have cleaned everything.

Sterilizing may not be absolutely necessary, but at the very minimum all your equipment should be dipped in boiling water, jars, jar lifter, lids, filters, funnels etc. To sterilize, boil for 10 minutes. Fresh out of the dishwasher would work also. Do not boil plastic containers.

Using a jar lifter will prevent burns, scalds, and dropping and breaking glass containers.

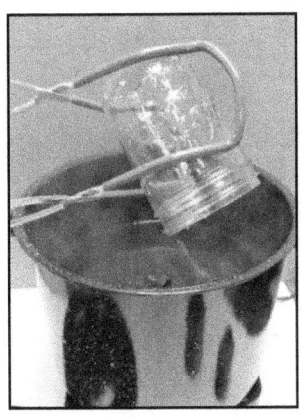

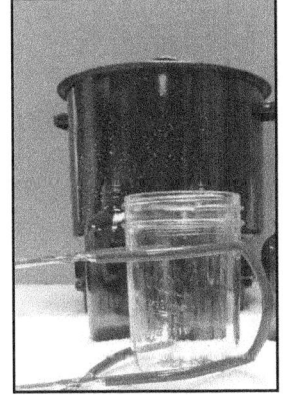

Setting jars right side up will allow the steam to escape and will dry your container.

Setting the container upside down will trap steam and allow moisture to remain.

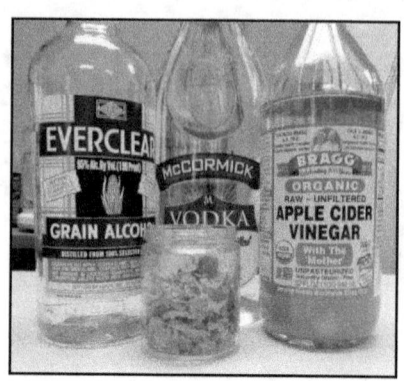

Chose your solvent, alcohol or vinegar.
Fill the jar half way with dried herbs.
If using fresh herbs, fill the jar all the way to the top with the fresh herbs and pack down.

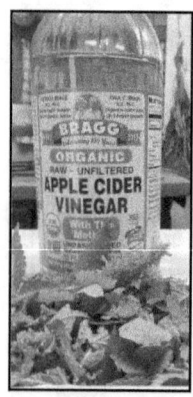

If using vinegar, warm up the vinegar for leaves and flowers. Bring to a boil for roots, bark and seeds.

Vinegar will corrode metal lids. Either use the plastic lids that are now available or place wax paper or plastic wrap between the jar and the lid.

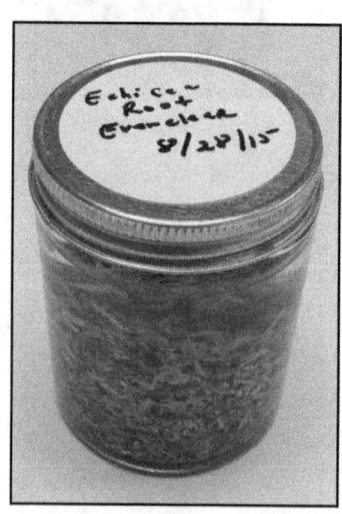

Fill the jar to the top with the solvent, Vodka, Everclear, or Vinegar.

Cap and label the tincture with the name of the herbs, solvent used and the date. Shake.

Shake daily for 2-6 weeks.

After a few hours, and after a few days, check and make sure the herbs are completely covered, adding more solvent if necessary.

STRAIN AND BOTTLING THE TINCTURES

Equipment: dark bottles, funnel, measuring cup, strainer (coffee filter, jelly bag or muslin.)
Choose your filter for straining.

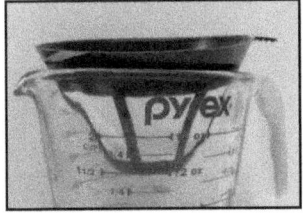

Re-usable coffee filter
Cone shaped best.

Or
Jelly bag with or without the coffee filter, or a muslin cloth.

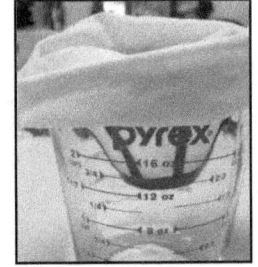

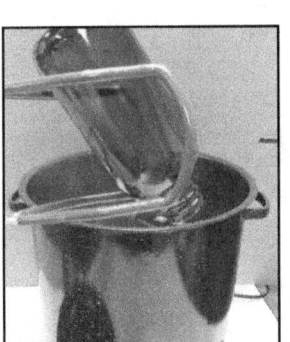

Dip all equipment, bottles, lids, staining filter, funnel, measuring cup, etc in boiling water or boil for 10 minutes.
Do not boil plastic containers.

Set out on a clean towel right side up.

The escaping steam from the boiling water will dry the equipment. Turning the containers upside down will trap the steam inside causing moisture.

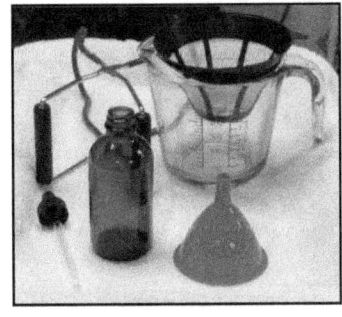

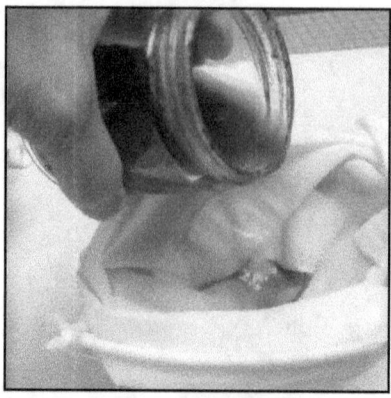

Pour tincture into measuring cup with strainer.

This may be just the coffee filter, or combined with the jelly bag, or muslin cloth.

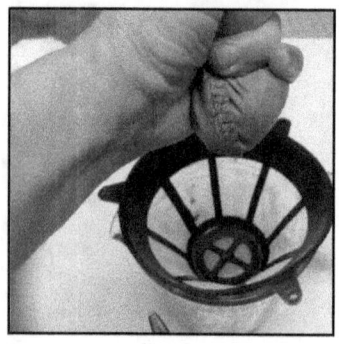

If using a jelly bag or muslin, squeeze out as much as you can.

If using the coffee filter, use a spoon and press against the filter to get ever last drop.

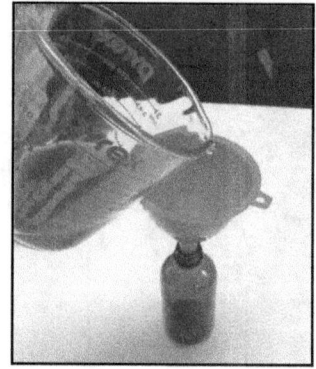

Pour into a dark bottle.
If you do not have dark bottles, a jar will work if you keep it in a dark place or cover it with a cloth.

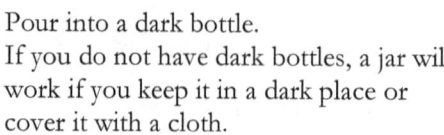

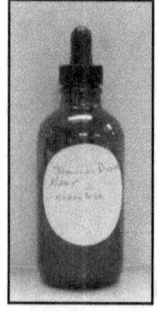

Label with the name of the herbs in the tincture, solvent used (Vodka, Everclear, Vinegar, Glycerin, etc. and date.

ECHNICEA ROOT AND SEED TINCTURE

Shelf life: Many years.

Dosage: 1/4 to ½ teaspoon every hour or at least several times a day at the first sign of cold or flu. When you know you have the cold or flu quit taking it. Begin again if you have an infection.

Although all parts of the plant can be used, different parts of the plant are harvested at different times of the year. Harvest the top part of the plant in the spring and summer. The roots and mature seeds would be harvested in the fall.

All parts stimulate the immune system. Only the root and seeds have a numbing effect.

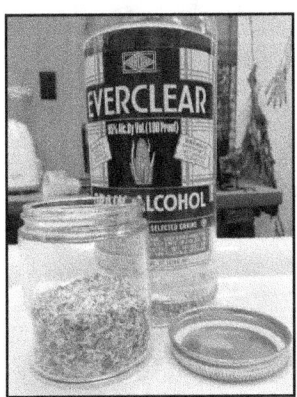

Begin with clean, preferred sterilized jar with tight fitting lid.

Chop the Echinacea Root, the smaller the pieces, the more of the medical properties will be extracted.

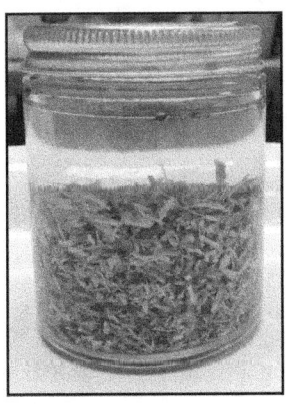

Fill the any size jar halfway with the Echinacea Root. Fill the jar to the top with the solvent. (Everclear preferred for roots, bark and seed) to completely cover the Echinacea Root .

Cap and label with the name of the herb, solvent used, and the date. Shake and then check in a few hours to make sure the herbs are completely covered.

Shake daily for 2-6 weeks.

Check in a few days to make sure the Echinacea Root is still completely covered, adding more alcohol if necessary.

Strain and Bottle

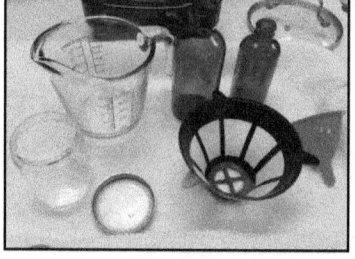

Begin with clean equipment and bottles.

Strain into your choice of a jelly bag, muslin cloth, or coffee filter.

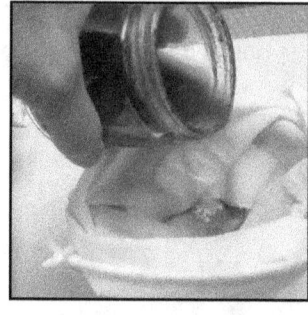

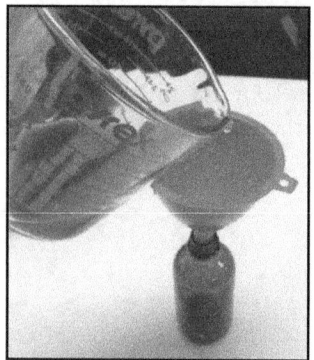

Pour into a dark bottle.
Cap and label with the name of the herb, solvent used, and the date.

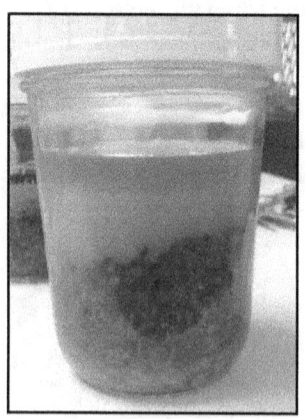

For the best of all the parts of the plant, harvest the tops in the spring and make the tincture, harvest the roots in the fall and make the tincture and combine the tinctures together.

Don't be alarmed if your Echinacea Root tincture becomes cloudy and separates. Roots and bark have resinous material that does not mix well with alcohol.

Always shake your tincture before you use it to combine the oils and alcohol.

ELDERBERRY TINCTURE

Simpler Method that will keep for many years.

Take 30-60 drops (1/4 to ½ teaspoon) every hour, or at least several times a day at the first sign of cold or flu.

Take 30-60 drops (1/4 to ½ teaspoon) up to 3 times a day as an antioxidant for eyesight.

Dried elderberries, chopped or crushed
Vodka or Everclear
Jar with tight fitting lid

Chop or crush dried elderberries. The finer the elderberries are chopped the more of the medical properties will be extracted.

Fill any size jar halfway with the chopped berries. Pour the solvent over the berries to the top of the jar. Cap and label. Shake.

Check in a few hours to make sure the elderberries are completely covered, adding more alcohol if necessary.

Shake daily for 2-6 weeks.

Check again in a few days to make sure the elderberries are completely covered, adding more alcohol if necessary.

Strain. Pour into dark bottle.

Label with the name of the herb, solvent used and the date.

Store in cool dark place.

SAGE TINCTURE

Dried Sage, chopped
Vodka or Everclear
Jar with tight fitting lid

Chop the Sage, the finer the chop the more of the medical properties will be extracted from the herb.

Fill any size jar halfway with chopped sage. Pour the solvent over the sage filling to the top of the jar. Cap and Label. Shake.

Check in a few hours to make sure the Sage is completely covered, adding more alcohol if necessary.

Shake daily for 2-6 weeks. Check again in a few days to make sure the Sage is completely covered, adding more alcohol if necessary.

Strain and pour into dark bottle and label with the name of the herb, the solvent used and the date.

Store in dark cool place.

SAGE AND ECHINACEA ROOT TINCTURE AS A GARGLE OR THROAT SPRAY

Combine equal amounts Sage Tincture and Echinacea Root tincture.

Add 5 ml (1 teaspoon) to 1 cup of warm water and gargle for a hot, swollen and painful throat

Combine equal amounts Sage and Echinacea Root Tinctures into a spray bottle and spray a hot, swollen and painful throat.

LEMON BALM PLUS TINCTURE

Use these same directions using 1 part Lemon Balm, 1 part Calendula, 1/2 part Licorice Root and 1/2 part St. John's Wort.

HERBAL ELIXARS

An herbal elixir is made by adding 1/4 part of food grade vegetable glycerin or honey to the formula. They are many recipes and formulas.

They are used to sweeten really bitter herbs such as hops to help make the medicine go down.

They can be used to soften tinctures made with Everclear that will burn your socks off when taken straight.

Example:
4 oz. of dried herb
2 oz. of food grade vegetable glycerin
6 oz. of Everclear

ELDERBERRY ELIXAR

Very long shelf life, take 1 tablespoon every hour at the first sign of a cold or flu, or take for coughs that produce a lot of mucus.

Dried elderberries
2 tablespoons of powdered ginger or 4 tablespoon of fresh grated ginger root.

Optional: Cinnamon sticks, Star Anise, Aniseed and cloves

Aniseed will act both as an expectorant (thins the mucus) and as an antispasmodic.

Fill a jar ½ full of the dried elderberries, add the ginger and the other herbs.

Cover the berries and other herbs with honey and stir.

Fill the jar to the top with Vodka.

Stir well.

Cap and label with the name of the herbs, solvents used and the date.

Shake daily for 2-6 weeks.

Strain and pour into bottle or jar.

Label with the name of the herbs, solvents used and the date.

ALCOHOL FREE TINCTURES: GLYCERITES

These may not be as potent and will not have the same shelf life (shelf life 2-3 years) as an alcohol based tincture but are better suited for children, the elderly or those that are very sensitive and those that cannot have alcohol. These will be more appropriate for applying to sensitive area.

Mix 3 parts food grade glycerin with 1 part of distilled water
Fill one jar ½ full of dried herb
Pour glycerin mixture to top of jar.
Cover with lid and shake 2 times daily for 4-6 weeks.
Strain and label jar.

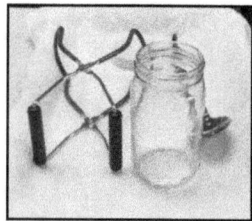

Begin with clean equipment. Either boil for 10 minutes to sterilize or at least dip into boiling water. Do not boil plastic containers.

Set out on clean towel right side up.

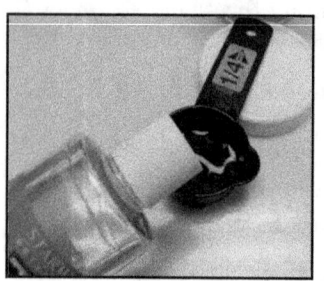

Mix 3 parts of food grade vegetable glycerin with one part of distilled water.

A part can be of any measurement such as 1/4 of a cup, ½ of a cup, etc.

Fill one jar half full of the dried herb.

Pour glycerin/water mixture to the top of the jar.

Cover the jar with a tight fitting lid. Label the jar with the name of the herbs, glycerin, and date.
Shake 2 times a day for 4-6 weeks.

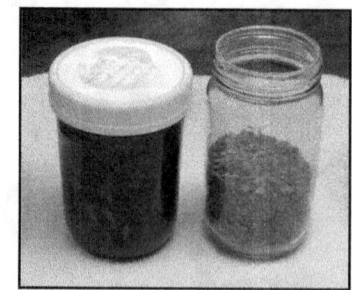

Strain and Label Your Product

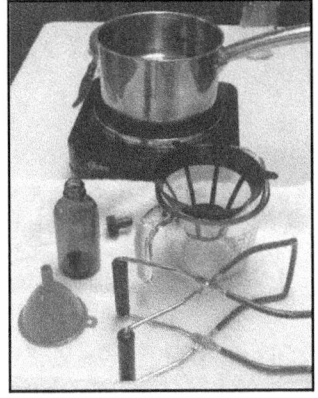

Sterilize or dip your equipment in boiling water and lay out on clean towel. Do not boil plastic containers.

Pour tincture into strainer.

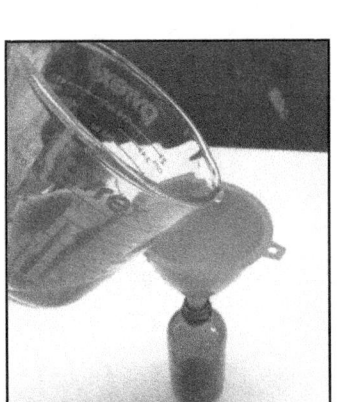

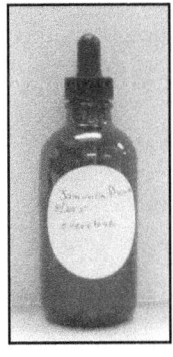

Pour strained tincture into dark bottle.

Label bottle with the name of the herbs, solvent and date.

Lemon Balm Plus makes an excellent Glycerite.

1 part Lemon Balm, 1 part Calendula, 1/2 part Licorice Root and 1/2 part St. John's Wort.

FLUID OR LIQUID EXTRACTS

These are commercially made products with specific weight and measurements and technical equipment and skills. These are made with alcohol and glycerin. Precise doses can be standardized to have a certain amount of the active ingredient. These are not homemade projects.

LINIMENTS

Liniments are made just like a tincture except made with rubbing alcohol and sometimes apple cider vinegar. How to make tinctures, pg. 91

I do not use rubbing alcohol, I use Vodka so that I can use the herbal remedy either way. This also prevents anyone from accidentally ingesting rubbing alcohol.

They can be used to stimulate muscles and ligaments or used to relax muscles and ligaments. If using rubbing alcohol, they are meant to go through the skin and never taken internally.

SYRUPS

Syrup can be as easy as adding 1 part tincture to 3 parts of a simple syrup mixture and store in the refrigerator.

Simple Syrup

To 1 pint of water add 2 ½ pounds of sugar. Stir to dissolve, bring to a boil and remove from heat.

Another method would be to add ¾ pounds of sugar to 1 pint of tincture and stir on low heat until the sugar is dissolved.

Honey Herbal Syrup

Add (1/4 cup) of dried herb or ½ cup of fresh herb to 1 quart (4 cups) of water. Boil down and reduce to 1 pint (2 cups)

Strain and add 2-4 tablespoons of honey. Store in the refrigerator for up to 1 month

ELDERBERRY SYRUP

Store in the refrigerator for about 2-4 weeks. Optional: Freeze in small containers allowing head room for the liquid to expand in the freezer. 1 tablespoon every hour or at least several times a day at the first sign of cold or flu, continue throughout the illness.

Take for coughs that produce a lot of mucus.

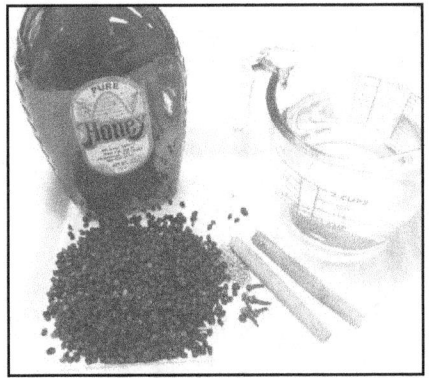

½ cup of dried elderberries Or 1 cup if using fresh or frozen elderberries 5 cloves ½ cinnamon sticks 2 cups of water (distilled preferred) 1 cup of water if using fresh elderberries Honey to taste Small saucepan with lid, muslin cloth or other strainer

Optional: 12 Star Anise or 1 teaspoon of Anise Seed. Star Anise and Anise Seed are different herbs. 1 tablespoon of grated fresh ginger or 1 teaspoon of the dried ginger powder 1 tablespoon of lemon juice

Anise Seed will act as both an expectorant (thins the mucus) and will help suppress the cough.

Note: According to a 2011 article in Alternative Medicine Studies, Star Anise is the primary source of shikimic acid, the precursor to oseltamivir, used in the anti-viral medication know as Tamiflu.

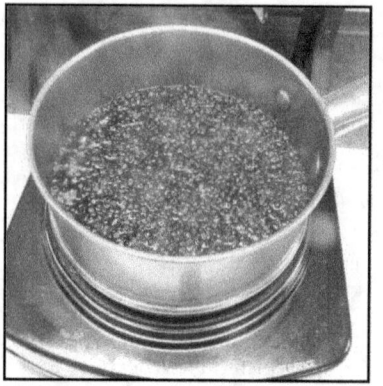

Combine the dried elderberries and other herbs with 2 cups of water, 1 cup of water if using fresh or frozen elderberries.

Cover the pan and bring to a boil and then simmer for about 20-30 minutes or until the liquid is reduced by half.

While the Elderberries are cooking, clean or sterilize the equipment and jars or bottles you will be using. Set out on a clean towel or surface.

Strain into a coffee filter, jelly bag or muslin cloth.

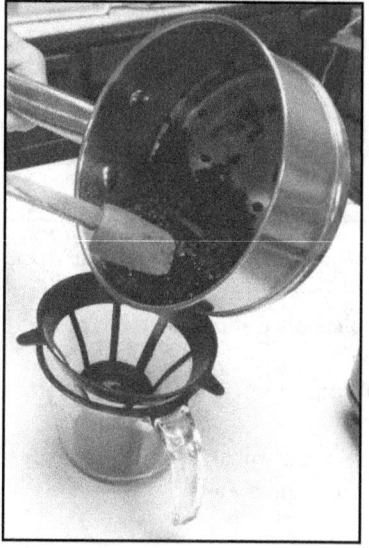

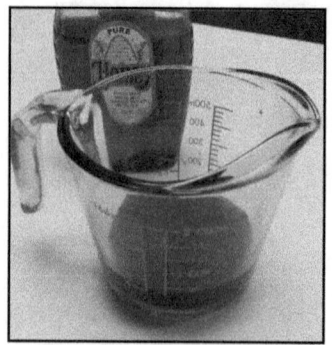

Add honey and lemon juice to taste.

The more honey that you use will preserve the syrup longer, up to equal amount of honey to liquid.

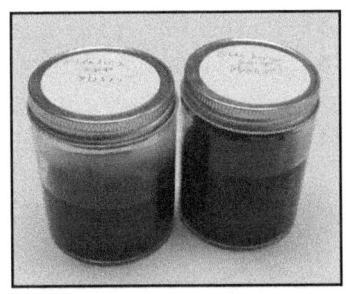

Pour into bottles or jars.
Label with the name of herbs and solvents
used and the date.

**For longer shelf life, use a recipe that is for canning Elderberry Jelly
and leave out the pectin for an Elderberry syrup with a long shelf.**

JUICING

Fruits and Vegetables that are juiced or blended.

POTHERBS

Herbs that are normally eaten as a food. Usually greens of some sort that
are cooked and eaten or used in salads.

SUPPOSITORIES

Suppositories are made with cocoa butter or other nut butter and mixed
with a finely powdered herb or they can be made with a mixture of gelatin,
glycerin and an herbal tincture or decoction.

INFUSED HERBAL OIL

Since all oils including herbal oils will go rancid, it is better to make in small batches and refrigerate, leaving out a small container at a time for personal use. Many herbalists soak the herbs in oil for 2-3 weeks in a sunny window. I prefer the heat method.

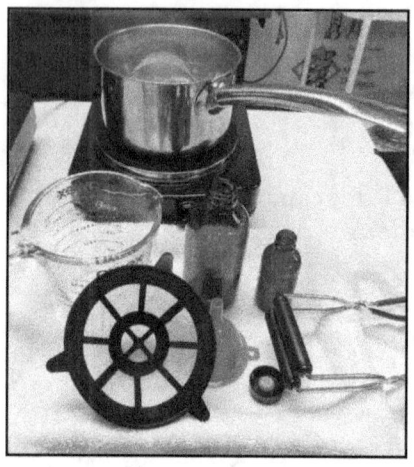

Use clean sterilized equipment. At the minimum dip your jars and bottles in hot boiling water. Do not boil plastic containers.

Placing bottles, lids, etc. right side up to allow escaping steam to dry bottles and equipment.

Place on clean towel or clean surface.

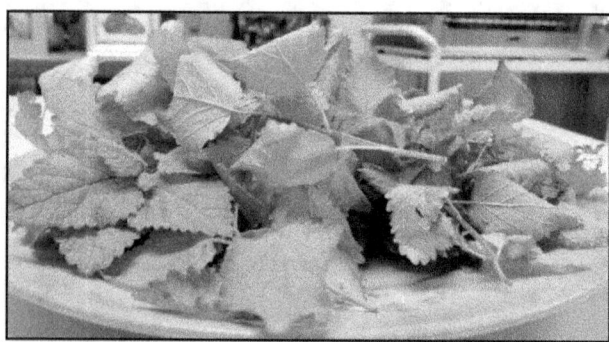

If using fresh herbs, let them wilt to remove some of the moisture. This could take an hour or ½ a day depending on the thickness of the herbs and how wet they were in the beginning.

Chop the herbs, (fresh or dried) the finer the herbs are chopped the more of the medical properties will be extracted.

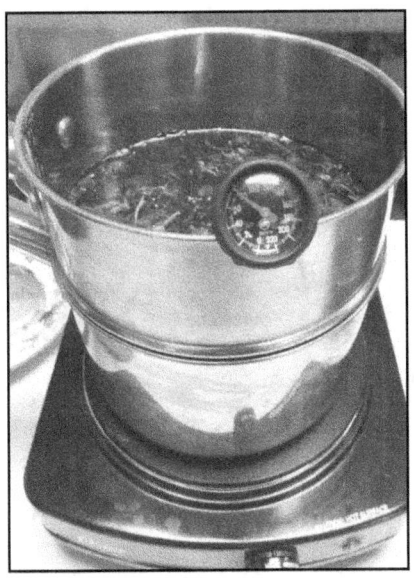

Place the prepared herbs into the double boiler, cover with 1-2 inches of your chosen oil.

Heat the oil keeping it below a simmer. Keep the temperature between 95°f - 110°f.

Heat gently for at least 1 hour. 2-3 hours would be even better. Overnight if you have the equipment to keep the oil between 95-110° f.

Dry the bottom of the pan on a towel to prevent hot water from dripping on you or your herbal remedy.

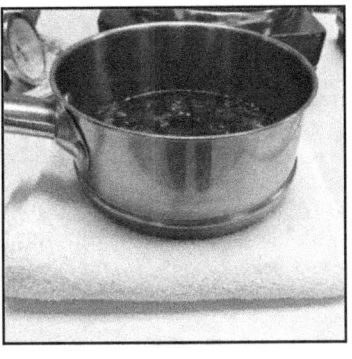

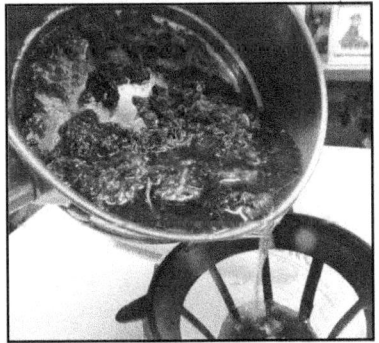

Strain the infused oil into the strainer of your choice. I prefer the plastic coffee filters.

I use a spoon to press the herbs against the filter to strain out as much of the oil as I can.

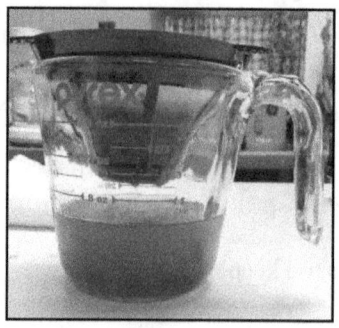

Adding a dropper full of Vitamin E to your strained oil will help preserve the infused oil.

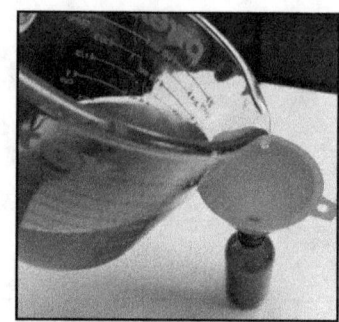

Pour into a clean dark bottle. A jar or a clear bottle can be used. A dark bottle or storing the remedy in a dark place will help preserve it longer.

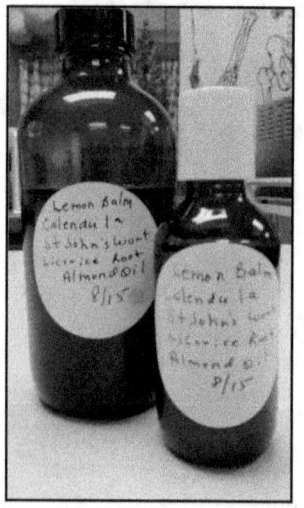

Label your jar or bottle with the herbs and the oil used and the date.

Other cooking methods.

An induction cook top would be great as you can set the temperature and the hours and leave it alone.

A yogurt maker would keep the oil at the perfect temperature.

OINTMENTS, SALVES, AND LIP BALMS

An ointment or salve begins with an infused herbal oil. The herbal oil is then thickened with beeswax. Approximately, 1 oz. (about 4 tablespoons) of beeswax per 8 oz. of herbal oil. Adding essential oils are optional. Most medical infused oils are made with a base of olive oil. Almond oil is best for the lips. Grapeseed oil is often used to make lotions. Our ancestors used whatever animal fat or vegetable oil that they had.

Although coconut oil is an awesome healing oil, it is normally combined with other oils to offset its property of turning into a liquid or solid state at various temperatures. There are countless recipes and methods using various combinations of oils. Making smaller amounts and using the smallest of containers is recommended because the ointment or salve can go rancid. The first time you stick your finger into a jar of salve or ointment, you have contaminated it, another reason to use the smallest of containers. Lip balms are really ointments or salves. If pouring into tubes you would use more beeswax.

If your remedy is too thin, reheat and use more beeswax. If you remedy is too hard, reheat and add more oil.

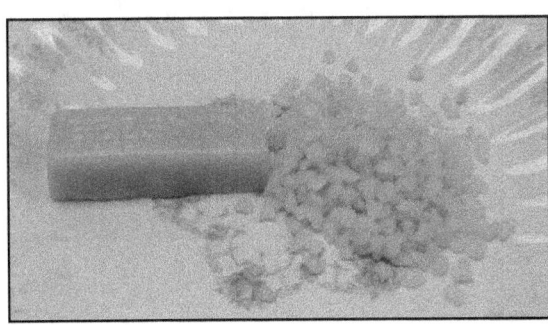

Beeswax comes in either a block form or in little beads called pastilles or pearls.

If you buy beeswax in a block, it is next to impossible to cut. You will first have to melt it down on low heat and then measure out the amount that you need.
The beeswax beads or pastilles is as simple as measuring or weighing the correct amount.

The following recipe can be doubled, tripled or halved. It is best to begin with small amounts before making larger recipes.

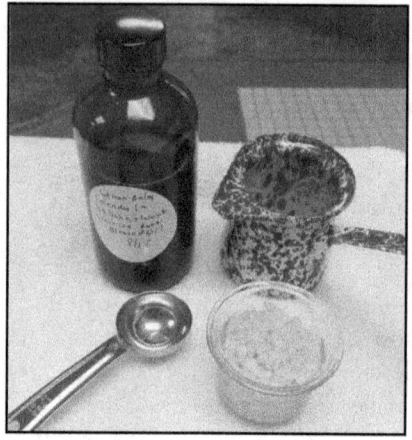

5 tablespoons of infused herbal oil
1 tablespoon of beeswax, 2 tablespoons if using the lip balm tubes.
Optional: 20 drops of essential oil
Makes 20 3 ml containers, or about 2 ½ oz.

I used 45 ml jars in this recipe and it made 2 jars.

Sterilize the jars and lids. At the minimum dip into boiling water.

Set out on clean towel or surface right side up so the escaping steam will quickly evaporate the water.

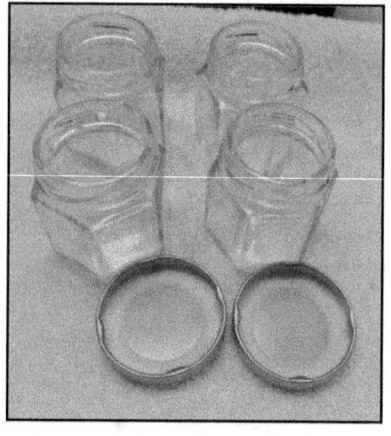

Setting the containers top down will trap the escaping steam keeping moisture in.

Moisture will cause bacteria growth in the ointment.

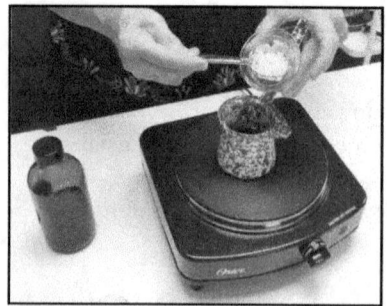

Heat 5 tablespoons of the infused herbal oil with 1 tablespoon of beeswax, (2 tablespoons if making lip balm in tubes) over very low heat until the beeswax is melted. Stir constantly.

Caution: beeswax is flammable.

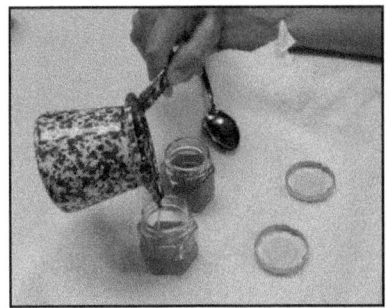

Pour into small containers.
If using essential oils wait 1 minute for the oil to cool slightly. Heat will make you essential oils evaporate.

Wipe out the pan you heated the oil and beeswax in to make clean up easier.

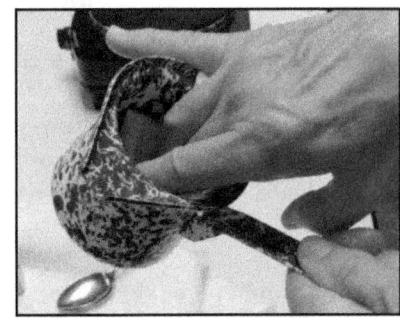

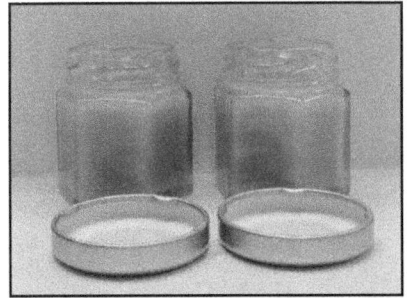

Let the ointment completely cool before putting on the lid to prevent condensation.

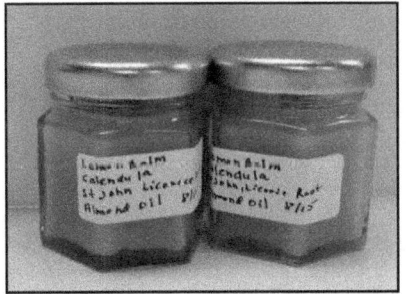

Cap the jar.

Clean the jar of any spills. Wiping the jar with alcohol will remove spilled oils and beeswax.

Label with name of the herbs and the oil used and the date.

LEMON BALM PLUS OIL

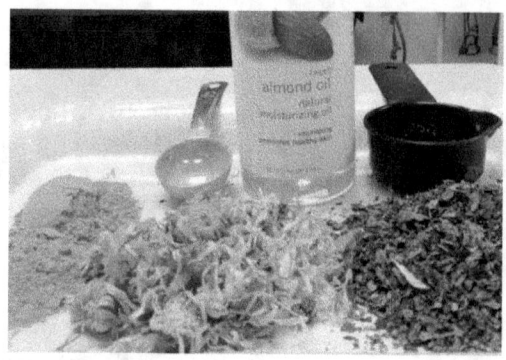

1 part chopped Lemon Balm (½ cup)
1 part Calendula (1/2 cup)
½ part St. John's Wort (1/4 cup) or (1 tablespoon if using powdered)
½ part Licorice Root (1/4 cup) or (1 tablespoon if using powdered)
Optional: Dropper full of Vitamin E
Almond Oil

Place herbs in top of a double boiler.

Cover the herbs with 1 to 2 inches of almond oil

Heat over very low heat.

Keep the heat around 95°f to 110°f 1 to 2 hours.

The longer the herbs are infused at the lowest heat will make the strongest herb oil. Even overnight if you have the equipment to keep the temperature around 95-110° f.

Dry the bottom of the pan on a towel to prevent the hot water from dripping on you or the herbal infusion.

Strain the infused oil into the strainer of your choice.

If using a jelly bag or muslin cloth twist the bag to extract as much of the oil that you can.

If using the coffee filter use a spoon or spatula to press against the filter to extract as much as you can.

Add a dropper full of vitamin E to help preserve the oil

Pour into clean, preferred sterilized dark bottle or jar.

Label with name of the herb, oil and the date.

LEMON BALM PLUS SALVE OR LIP BALM

5 tablespoons of the Lemon Balm Plus Oil

1 tablespoon of beeswax, 2 tablespoon if making lip balm for the tubes

Optional: 20 drops of essential oil.

Makes 20 3 ml containers, about 2 ½ oz.

Heat 5 tablespoons of the infused oil with 1 tablespoon of beeswax over very low heat, stirring constantly until the beeswax is melted.

Caution: beeswax is flammable.

Pour into small containers.

If using essential oils, wait 1 minute for the oil to cool slightly. Essential oils will evaporate in heat.

Let the salve cool completely before putting on the lid to prevent condensation.

Clean the jar of any spills. Wiping the jar with alcohol will remove spilled oils and beeswax.

Label with the name of the herbs, oil used and essential oils if used and the date.

Larger Amounts:
1 cup of Lemon Balm Plus Oil mix with 1 oz. (about 4 tablespoons) of Beeswax.

ALL PURPOSE HEALING SALVE

There are countless recipes, ever herbalist has their favorite.
Most healing salves will have a combination of Comfrey with Calendula,
and maybe add Plantain and Chickweed or maybe St. John's Wort.
Your all purpose healing salve can be just 2 herbs, 5 herbs, any number of
herbs. If using Comfrey combine it either with Calendula or Echinacea.
Comfrey regenerates cell growth but is not an antiseptic. Comfrey alone
could cause skin to grow over an infection. Calendula regenerates cell
growth but is also an antiseptic. Echinacea fights infections.

Your all purpose salve could be Comfrey combined with Echinacea, or it
could be Comfrey combined with Calendula, or Plantain combined with
Calendula.

There are so many choices that allow you to use what you have on hand.
My favorite is the recipe from Rosemary Gladstar.
1 part Comfrey
1 part Calendula
1 part St. John's Wort

Follow the directions for making an herbal oil and salve.

Make herbal oil using
1 cup of dried herbs
12 oz. of oil
Add 1 oz. of beeswax to make salve.

OXYMELS # 1

Oxymels are basically your herb of choice, vinegar and honey.

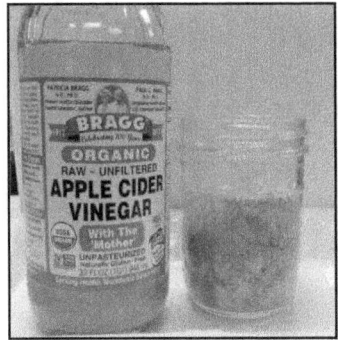

Fill any size jar 1/3 to ½ full of chopped or minced herb.

Fill the jar 2/3 full of apple cider vinegar.

If using a pint jar that would be 4 oz. of the chopped herb and 6 oz. of vinegar.

Fill the jar to the top with honey.

If using a pint jar that would be 6oz. of honey.

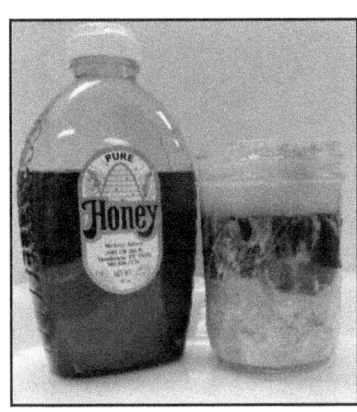

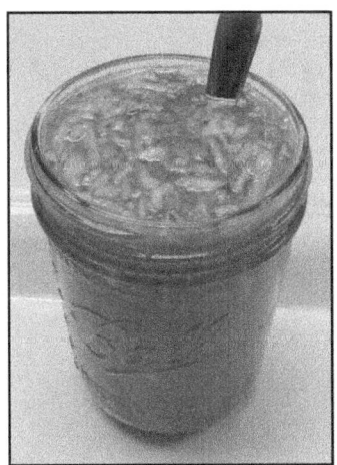

Stir the herb, vinegar and honey mixture.

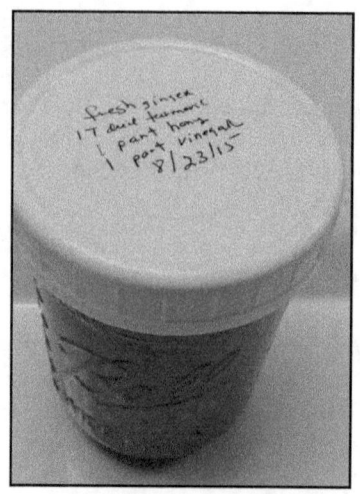

Cap and label with the name of the herbs, solvent (vinegar), and date.

Shake each day for 2-6 weeks.

You may need to add more vinegar and honey if the herbs do not remain covered.

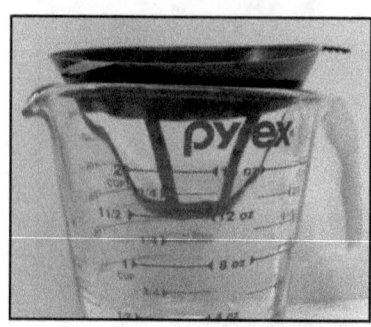

Strain and pour into bottle or jar.

Label with the name of the Oxymel and date.

Oxymels will keep for many months, for longer storage, keep in the refrigerator.

Take by the spoonful or add to hot water and drink as a tea or use as the base for marinades and dressings.

OXYMELS # 2

Take any herbal vinegar and add honey to taste.

GINGER OXYMEL

This will keep for many months, for longer storage, keep in the refrigerator.
Take by the spoonful or add to hot water to drink as a hot tea.
Take as an immune builder and to help thin mucus.
Ginger is a mild anti-inflammatory. Adding the optional Turmeric will boost this effect.

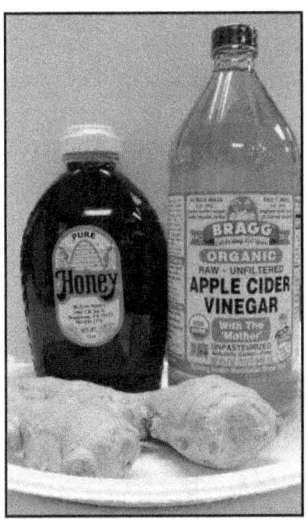

1 part fresh Ginger Root, grated or minced
Optional: Add a tablespoon of dried Turmeric.
1 part Apple Cider Vinegar
1 part honey

For a pint jar:
4 oz. or grated Ginger Root
6 oz. of honey
6 oz. of Apple Cider Vinegar

Grate of mince ginger root. Caution: be careful with grater not to cut your fingers.
Fill jar 1/4 to 1/3 full.
Fill jar 2/3 full of Apple Cider Vinegar.
Stir the Ginger Root and Vinegar.
Fill the top of the jar with honey.
Stir well.
Cap and label with the name of herbs, solvents used and the date.
Shake each day for 2-4 weeks.
Strain and pour into another jar or bottle.
Cap, and label with the name of the herbs, solvents used and the date.

SLIPPERY ELM THROAT AND TUMMY SOOTHERS

Although many herbalists will call these lozenges I do not because the first thing one thinks of are the hard candy cough drops. I could have given you recipes for those type but then it would not be easy for beginners. These throat soothers are formed from dried powdered herbs, Licorice Root tea and honey and some have the addition of essential oils. They are dried and stored in the refrigerator for the longest shelf life. They are meant to be sucked on so that the mucilage will soothe and moisten your throat by coating it. If they were not dried they would immediately dissolve in your mouth and then they wouldn't be doing their job. A few can be carried around in a tin in your purse or pocket to be used as needed.

Marshmallow root or Plantain could be used but I prefer the Slippery Elm. Marshmallow Root has a distinct aroma and taste which I suppose some herbalists just love, but I guess it is an acquired taste that I have not acquired. Other herbal teas can be used instead of Licorice Root tea. Licorice Root adds that extra sweetness along with a flavor many are familiar with. It has antiviral properties and is a demulcent.
Molasses can be used instead of honey.
These recipes are a base from which you can get started with and then create and adjust for your own individual taste and needs.

All these recipes begin with a strong Licorice Root Tea:
1 teaspoon of chopped dried Licorice Root or 1/2 teaspoon of powdered
1/2 cup of water
Make a strong Licorice Root tea by simmering 1/2 cup water with the Licorice Root.
Simmer covered 10-15 minutes until the tea is reduced to 1/4 cup.

BASIC SLIPPERY ELM THROAT SOOTHER OR TUMMY SOOTHER

4 teaspoons of the strong Licorice Root tea pg. 122
2 tablespoon of Slippery Elm Powder divided plus extra for rolling
1 tablespoon of honey
Small bowl or plate
Wax or parchment paper
Upside down paper plate
Rolling pin

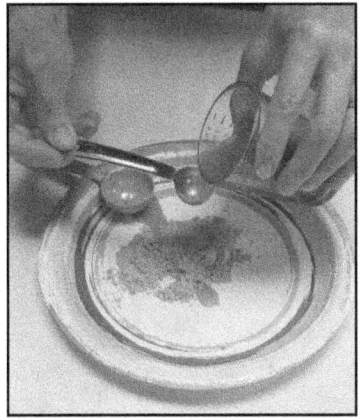

Place 1 tablespoon of the Slippery Elm Powder in a bowl or small plate.

Stir in 1 teaspoon of the Licorice Root tea into the Slippery Elm Powder.

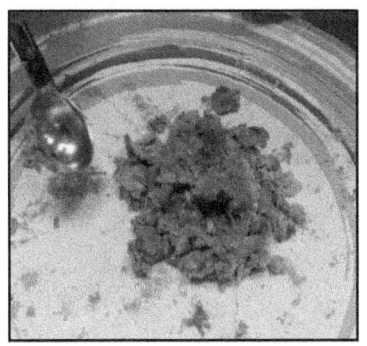

Continue to stir in the other 3 teaspoons of Licorice Root tea until thoroughly moistened.

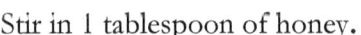

Stir in 1 tablespoon of honey.

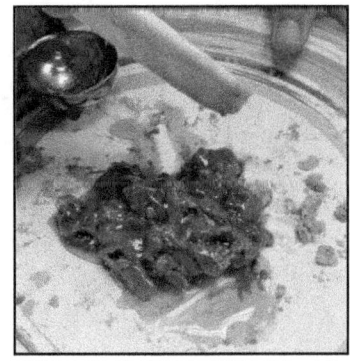

123

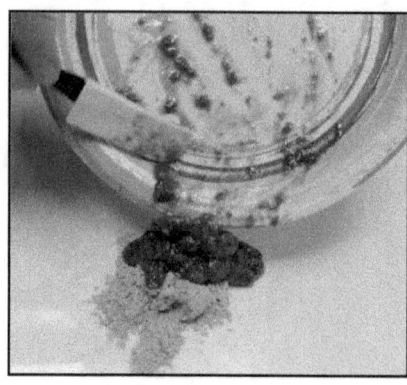

Lay wax paper or parchment paper on table.

Place 1 tablespoon of Slippery Elm powder on the paper.

Pour honey mixture over the Slippery Elm powder.

Mix all ingredients together.

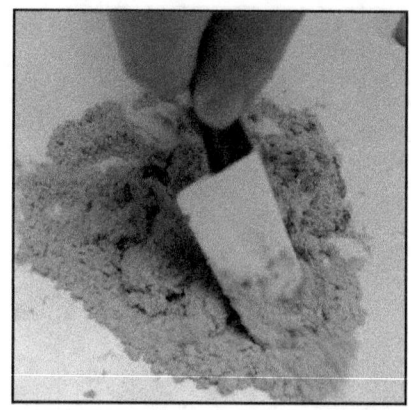

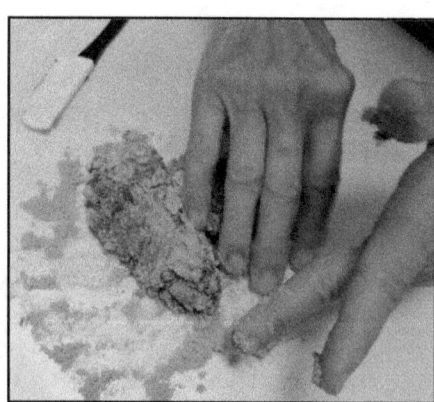

Continue to mix the mixture with your hands, forming into a ball like you would a pie crust.

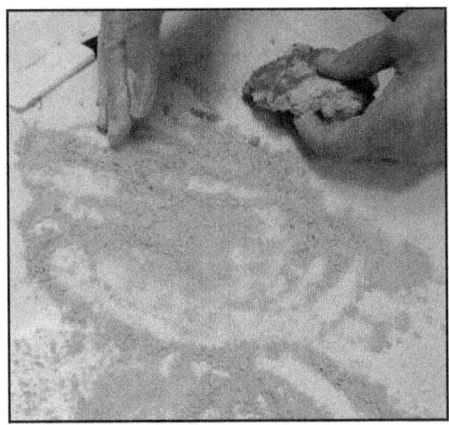

Sprinkle additional Slippery Elm powder onto the wax paper and dust the rolling pin with the Slippery Elm powder.

Roll out about 1/4 inch thick. Add more Slippery Elm powder if needed.

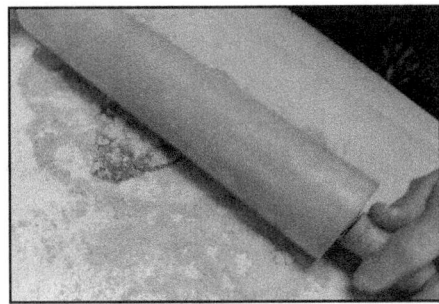

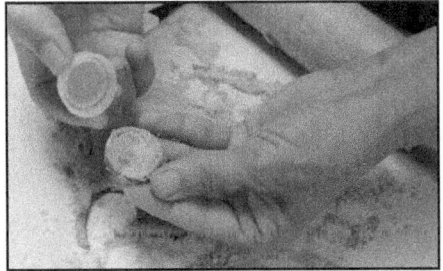

Use bottle cap to cut into small circles.
If you do not have that kind of patience,

Use a knife or a pizza cutter to cut into small squares.
Keep in mind what size would be comfortable in your mouth.

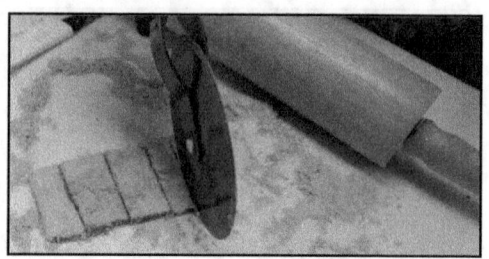

Dry on a paper plate turned upside down.
Turn each day until completely dry.
A dehydrator or an oven with a light bulb could be used.

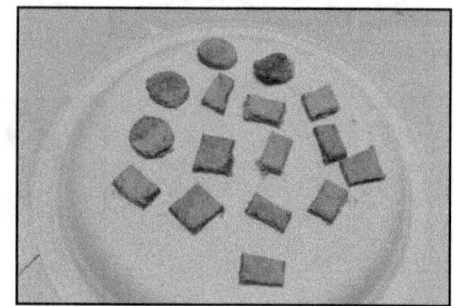

These are meant to be sucked on. A mucilage gel will form, continuously coating your irritated throat.

If you use these before they dry, they will dissolve immediately, not functioning as a lozenge.

Store in a plastic bag or small jar in the refrigerator. Keep a small amount in your purse to use when that little irritating cough occurs or to stop the constant clearing in your throat.

Once you have mastered this basic recipe, there are numerous variations.

GINGER THROAT SOOTHER OR TUMMY SOOTHER

4-5 teaspoons of the Strong Licorice Root tea pg. 122
4 teaspoons of Slippery Elm powder plus 2 teaspoon of Ginger Root powder mixed together, divided, extra Slippery Elm Powder and Ginger for rolling.
1 tablespoon of honey
Optional: 1 drop of essential oil of Lemon

Place 1 tablespoon of the Slippery Elm Powder/Ginger Root powder in a bowl or small plate.
Stir in 1 teaspoon of the Licorice Root tea into the Slippery Elm/Ginger Root powder continuing to add 1 teaspoon at a time to completely moisten the Slippery Elm/Ginger Root powder. Optional: Mix in the 1 drop of essential oil of Lemon.
Stir in the 1 tablespoon of honey and knead into a dough.
Lay Wax Paper or Parchment paper on the table.
Put 1 tablespoon of the Slippery Elm/Ginger on the paper.
Stir in the honey mixture with the Slippery Elm/Ginger powder and form into a patty.
Sprinkle Slippery Elm/Ginger Powder on the wax paper or parchment paper.
Sprinkle a little of the powder on the rolling pin.
Roll out about 1/4 inch thick. Add more powder if needed.
Either cut into small circles with a small cap or cut into squares with a knife or pizza cutter, depending on how much patience you have.
Place on top of an upside down paper plate to dry.
Or place in a food dehydrator or the oven with only the light bulb on to dry.
Turn each day to dry.
Label and store in a plastic bag, small tin, or small jar.

These are spicy!

PEPPERMINT PATTY

4 teaspoons of the strong Licorice Root tea pg. 122
1 tablespoon of Slippery Elm Powder
1 tablespoon of honey
1-2 drops of essential oil of Peppermint
2 teaspoons of cocoa plus 1 teaspoon of Slippery Elm powder mixed together plus extra for rolling
Wax or parchment paper
Upside down paper plate
Rolling pin

Place 1 tablespoon of the Slippery Elm Powder in a bowl or small plate.
Stir in 1 teaspoon of the Licorice Root tea into the Slippery Elm powder continuing to add 1 teaspoon at a time to completely moisten the Slippery Elm powder.
Stir in the 1 tablespoon of honey and knead into a dough.
Stir in the 1-2 drops of essential oil of Peppermint.
Lay out wax paper or parchment paper on the table.
Put the Slippery Elm/Cocoa Powder on the paper.
Mix in the honey mixture, knead into a small patty.
Sprinkle the additional Cocoa/Slippery Elm powder on the wax or parchment paper.
Sprinkle a little of the powder on the rolling pin.
Roll out about 1/4 inch thick. Add more powder as needed.
Either cut into small circles with a small cap or cut into squares with a knife or pizza cutter, depending on how much patience you have.
Place on top of an upside down paper plate to dry.
Or place in a food dehydrator or the oven with only the light bulb on to dry.
Turn each day to dry.
Label and store in a plastic bag, small tin, or small jar.

When using essential oils store in either a glass or metal container. The essential oils will evaporate through a plastic bag.

CINNAMON GINGER

4-5 teaspoons of the strong Licorice Root tea
1 tablespoon of Slippery Elm Powder plus 1 teaspoon of Ginger Root powder mixed together.
1 tablespoon of honey
1 tablespoon of Cinnamon powder plus extra as needed
Wax or parchment paper
Upside down paper plate
Rolling pin

Place 1 tablespoon of the Slippery Elm Powder/Ginger in a bowl or small plate.
Stir in 1 teaspoons of the Licorice Root tea into the Slippery Elm/Ginger powder continuing to add 1 teaspoon at a time to completely moisten the Slippery Elm powder.
Stir in the 1 tablespoon of honey and knead into a dough.
Lay out wax paper or parchment paper on the table.
Place the 1 tablespoon of Cinnamon powder on the paper.
Stir in the honey mixture and knead into a patty.
Sprinkle the remaining Cinnamon powder on the wax or parchment paper.
Sprinkle a little of the powder on the rolling pin. Roll out about 1/4 inch thick. Add more powder as needed.
Either cut into small circles with a small cap or cut into squares with a knife, depending on how much patience you have.
Place on top of an upside down paper plate to dry. Or place in a food dehydrator or the oven with only the light bulb on to dry.
Turn each day to dry.
Label and store in a plastic bag, small tin, or small jar.

These are spicy!

ESSENTIAL OILS

Essential Oils are distilled herbs or flowers. This is the concentrated essence of the plant. Citrus oils are pressed from the skin of the fruit, orange, grapefruit, lemon or lime. Jasmine is not an essential oil but an absolute. Absolutes use chemical extraction, so know your source and the chemical used during extraction before using therapeutically. Essential oils are also made from distilling tree resin such as Frankincense and Myrrh.

Aromatherapy uses these concentrated essences as an alternative therapy to promote the body's natural healing process to achieve balance and harmony. As essential oils evaporate they are inhaled, entering the body through the millions of cells that line the nasal passages effecting the body's psychological well being through the limbic system. Information from what we smell is sent to specific areas of the brain that influence memory, learning, basic emotions, hormonal balances and the flight or fight response. When essential oils are mixed with oils and lotions and massaged into the skin their tiny molecule structure allow them to penetrate the skin affecting the body physically. The fats that are used as carrier oils lie on the skin surface.

The Chinese were probably the first to discover the medical power of plants around 4500 B.C., but the Egyptians refined the art. All major civilizations and religions used essential oils.

The term "Aromatherapy" was termed in 1928 by the French chemist René Maurice Gatteforsse to describe the therapeutic action of essential oils.

Essential oils are very concentrated so they are used by drops. They normally are not taken orally but used instead by either inhalation are being diluted with lotions and massaged into the skin depending on the treatment required. You can buy a diffuser to diffuse the oil or use a cool mist humidifier. I personally don't like heat diffusion, but that is a matter of personal preference. Heat will destroy part of the medical benefits.

Everyone knows the benefits of using Eucalyptus and Peppermint for respiratory ailments and pain relief. A mixture of Eucalyptus and Peppermint can be rubbed on the temples or forehead for some types headaches. Basil can be used for some types of headaches. Lavender is good for tension type headaches. Generally if over the counter pain relievers help your headaches these oils will work. If you have the type headache that do not respond to pain medication these essential oils will probably not work either.

Research by Dr. Dembar of the University of Cincinnati showed that inhaling Peppermint oil increased the mental accuracy of students by 28%. Rosemary is also good for memory.

Rose scented oils and Citrus oils are uplifting. Lavender is calming.

Nearly all essential oils have anti-bacterial qualities. Lemon oil is used in many European hospitals as an antiseptic instead of chemicals. The main benefit of using essential oils are that bacteria and virus do not mutate to essential oils as they mutate to chemicals.

Research now indicates that essential oils may be the drug of the future to aid in treating emotional and mental disorders. In 1989 it was discovered that the amygdala (a gland of the brain) plays a major role in storing and releasing emotional trauma. Only odor or fragrance stimulation has a profound effect in triggering a response with this gland.

Certain essential oils, do not cover up odors in your home but will **actually break the odors down and eliminate the offending odor. Synthetic oils cannot do this.**

Diffusing some oils in your home will help eliminate airborne bacteria. Tea Tree oil is used for fungal infections.

We experience aromatherapy everyday of our lives. We smell bread baking or charcoal and lighter fluid and we get hungry. A lady wearing perfume passing by may make us feel pleasant or give us a headache. A skunk or a rotting dead animal may make us feel nauseated. Real Estate agents may burn a candle with the scent of chocolate chips cookies to give the property a feeling of home. Detailers give a used car that final touch with a new car scent.

Aromas can bring back memories. As a young wife back in the seventies a friend brought over fresh baked yeast bread. I instantly did not like the smell of the bread. I now realize it was because I spent 3 years in Buckner

Baptist Children's Home where they had their own bakery. Each day the smell of yeast bread baking circulated around the entire campus. At the time I did not know why I disliked the smell of the bread , but it still effected me. I now love yeast bread.

Have you heard the saying, Pine- Sol clean? Back in my day, the only cleaning products were Pine- Sol and Lysol.

When I smell the original Lysol scent I think of Buckner Baptist Children's Home. We used Lysol there. When I smell Pine- Sol, I think of home because that is what my mother cleaned with.

My first husband was injured in Viet Nam and spent 17 months in the hospital at Fort Sam Houston. Later he could not enter a hospital to visit family or friends because the scent of a hospital made him sick. He later died in a construction accident.

Essential oils can affect us through inhalation or being massage into the skin.

The same essential oil can have one effect when it is being inhaled and a different affect when it is massaged into the skin.

Peppermint or camphor will open up sinus when inhaled. But you can inhale it all you want and it will not have an analgesic effect on sore muscles until it is massaged into the skin.

Most essential oils have very subtle effects. Do not expect that a one-time application of essential oils or herbs are going to magically relieve depression, stop tension or even relieve insomnia. They must be used repeatedly throughout the day. They will enhance the ritual of taking a bath or preparing a cup of tea. They will make a massage more effective. Remember they help bring balance. You must also work on the cause. If you are royally pissed off, or just experienced a knock down, drug out fight, there is no herb or essential oil that is going to bring you peace and calm.

You can see more immediate results from the more aggressive essential oils that contain menthol for their cooling effect on pain, or Eucalyptus or Peppermint for sinus decongestion. An extract of Cayenne will have an immediate heating action. Ginger or Peppermint tea may bring quick relief from indigestion or nausea.

It takes 1 acre to make 15-20 pounds of Lavender oil. It takes 60,000 roses to make one ounce of rose oil which makes rose oil the most expensive essential oil you can buy. Essential oils may seem expensive for such tiny bottles, but remember they are concentrated so you only need a few drops at a time.

Use essential oils with caution. Most essential oils cannot be applied directly to the skin but must be diluted with oils, lotions and other carriers. The few exceptions to this are Lavender and Tea Tree. Essential oils may take the finish off of furniture. Keep the bottles away from children. Lavender and Tea Tree may be safe for children in diluted amounts. Even though Lavender and Tea Tree oil are safe for children my grandchild will tell you that Lavender Oil burns. People can be allergic to certain essential oils just as they are allergic to plants in nature. If you are allergic to cedar trees you are certainly allergic to cedar oil.

Essential oils and fragrant oils are not the same. Fragrances are usually synthetic oil and may cause allergies. Essential oils will state 100 % essential oil on the bottle. If it does not say 100% essential oil it could be a carrier oil with essential oils added to it, or just synthetic fragrances. Fragrant oils or synthetic oils have more varieties to choose from, can many times be more pleasant than essential oils and their fragrance will last much longer than essential oils. Certified Aroma Therapists will argue that a synthetic fragrance cannot be Aroma Therapy. But I point out if that fragrance affects you emotionally is that not aroma therapy? It certainly cannot have a physical effect. But it can have a psychological effect.

All plants do not have essential oils.

Examples of synthetic oils.

Apple, Carnation, Coconut, Lilac, Peach, Rain, Raspberry, Strawberry, Rose that costs less than $50 for 2 ml.

9 Additional Recipes

GARLIC

When using garlic to fight the cold or flu use fresh.

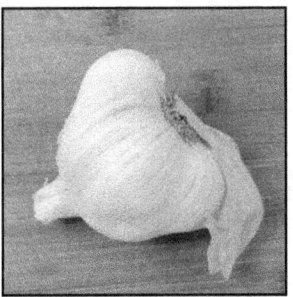

Garlic is considered nature's antibiotic. Of course most know that a cold or flu is not a bacteria so it will not respond to antibiotics. Garlic like most herbs are not an antibiotic, they are antimicrobial which means virus, fungus or bacteria.

When using garlic as an antibiotic or antimicrobial mince the garlic and let it set 10-15 minutes. The garlic cells must be ruptured to release two separate chemicals of the garlic, alliin and alliinase which then form a new compound called allicin.

Eating too much garlic at once may cause tummy problems, so start slowly and build up.

GARLIC AND HONEY

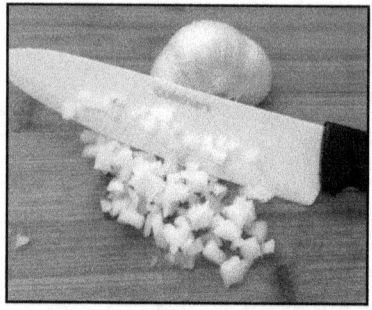

Mince 3-5 cloves of garlic. Let set 10-15 minutes.

Optional: Use a garlic press.

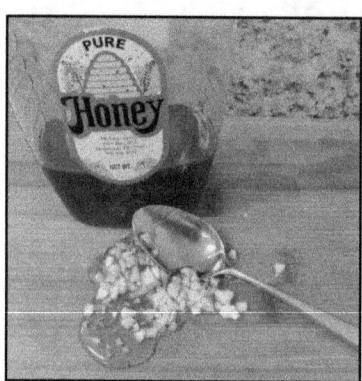

Place 1 tablespoon of honey on a plate.
Optional: Mix in 1/8 teaspoon (or a pinch) of powdered cayenne pepper.

Add the minced garlic to the honey mixture.

The honey will stick to the throat, the cayenne pepper increases circulation and the garlic stimulates the immune system.
Take a spoonful once an hour or at least 3-4 times a day.

GARLIC BUTTER

Mince the garlic and let set 10-15 minutes.
Add butter or olive oil.
As a base start with 2 parts butter or olive oil to 1 part minced garlic. Adjust from there.
If your tummy can handle more garlic use more, if not use less.
Spread on bread and eat throughout the day. Do not cook the garlic. If you want hot bread, heat the bread first and then spread the garlic and oil onto the hot bread.

GARLIC CIDER VINEGAR

There are many variations of this recipe. The main ingredients are the cloves of garlic, peppers and apple cider vinegar. If you are using horseradish the cooler months are the only time fresh horseradish is available. Anti viral herbs are then added. Use what you have, do not let the lack of the other ingredients keep you from making Garlic Cider Vinegar.

10 cloves of garlic, minced let set 10-15 minutes.
½ cup grated or chopped ginger
½ cup grated horseradish
1 medium chopped onion
2 chopped jalapeno or cayenne peppers
Zest and juice of 1 lemon
Several sprigs of rosemary
1 tablespoon of powdered turmeric or 1/4 cup of fresh grated turmeric root
Optional spices such as cinnamon and cloves. (The spice Clove buds, not more cloves of Garlic.

Combine in a quart jar. Some recipes say heat the vinegar, others say do not. If you are using regular store bought pasteurized vinegar, there are no living enzymes to kill. If you are using unpasteurized organic apple cider vinegar with the mother do not heat so as not to kill the enzymes. Heat apple cider vinegar until warm, do not boil or over heat, you do not want to kill the enzymes. Add the apple cider vinegar to the jar and cover with a plastic lid. If you only have a metal lid place a piece of plastic wrap between the lid and the jar to prevent the vinegar from corroding the lid.

Store in a cool dark place for 1 month, shaking daily. Strain and then add 1/4 cup of honey or to taste.

Take a spoonful at a time at the first sign of a cold or continue to take once you become sick. This can also be used to make an oil and vinegar dressing or vegetable marinades.

Garlic Cider Vinegar Dressing or Marinade
1/4 cup of Garlic Cider Vinegar
1/4 cup olive oil
2 tablespoons of spicy southwest ground mustard or other mustard of your choice. Mustard not only adds flavor but also acts as an emulsifier.

GINGER TEA

Fresh Ginger:
1 inch piece of ginger grated or chopped
Lemon juice to taste or vinegar
Honey to taste
Optional: pinch of cayenne pepper
8 oz. of boiling water.

Combine and steep covered 10-15 minutes. Strain and add honey and lemon juice to taste.
Drink throughout the day.

Iced Ginger Tea (Ginger ale) Add cold water and ice. If you have sparkling water that would be a nice touch.

Dried Ginger
2 teaspoons of Ginger powder
Lemon juice to taste or vinegar
Honey to taste
Optional: pinch of cayenne pepper
10 oz. of water.
Bring the water and ginger powder to a boil and simmer covered for 7 minutes. Strain and add honey and lemon to taste.
Drink throughout the day.

Note: Roots are normally brought to a boil and simmered (decoction) fresh Ginger roots are an exception. Steep fresh Ginger Root, simmer dried Ginger Root.

GINGER SMOOTHIE

Orange juice, oranges, fresh Ginger root and optional wheatgrass powder or other green powder, add honey for sweetness.

SAGE AND THYME VINEGAR

1 oz. of ground Sage leaves
1 oz. of ground Thyme leaves
1 qt. of apple cider vinegar
Honey to taste would be optional

Place herbs in a quart jar, heat apple cider vinegar until just warm, do not boil or overheat as not to destroy enzymes, and pour over the herbs. Let set for 14 days, shaking each day. Strain and pour into a dark bottle. Dilute into warm water and use as a mouthwash, a gargle or throat spray.

CHICKEN SOUP STEEPED WITH SAGE AND THYME

Open a can of chicken noodle or rice soup. Bring to a boil, turn off heat and add 1/2 to 1 teaspoon of Sage, Thyme and Black Pepper. Optional, add a little garlic. Or 1 spring or Sage and Thyme.
Cover and steep for 10 minutes.

EASY CHICKEN TORTILLA SOUP

1 qt of chicken broth
1 can of diced tomatoes and green chilies (Rotel)
Canned chicken
Optional: 2-4 chicken bouillon cubes according to how salty the chicken broth is.
1/2 teaspoon to 1 teaspoon of Sage and Thyme, or 1 fresh spring of Thyme and Sage and Black Pepper. Optional: a little Garlic
Bring the chicken stock, chicken, diced tomatoes and green chilies to a boil. Turn off heat, add the herbs, cover and steep for 10 minutes.
Serve over rice. Optional: Serve with Corn tortilla chips, cheese and avocado.

BEST CHICKEN TORTILLA SOUP

1 whole chicken
1 carrot
1 onion
Garlic
2 tablespoons of apple cider vinegar
Crock pot
Diced tomatoes and green chilies (Rotel)
2-4 chicken bouillon cubes
1/2-1 teaspoon of Sage and Thyme, or 1 sprig of Sage and Thyme, Black Pepper

Place chicken, carrots and onions, garlic and the 2 tablespoons of apple cider vinegar in a crock pot and cook overnight in the crock pot.
Bone the chicken and add back in as much chicken as you want.
Add the can of diced tomatoes and green chilies, chicken bouillon cubes according to how salty you like it.
Bring to a boil, turn off heat. Add the Sage and Thyme and Black Pepper. Cover and steep 10 minutes.
Serve over rice.   Optional: Serve with Corn tortilla chips, cheese and avocado

10 Herb Library

This is not meant to be a complete description of these herbs, nor give all of the medical properties or cautions. There is no herb book that will have all herbs in it. David Hoffman's books are a good source.

BLACK COHOSH

Acatea racemose,
Former name, Cimicfuga racemosa
Part used: rhizome and roots

Pain: Anti-inflammatory and muscle relaxer, Rheumatic arthritis, nerve pain, back pain, headaches

Muscle relaxer: Stop occasional muscle spasms, usually works within the hour. Not effective for chronic back pain.

Contraindications: do not use if pregnant, nursing or have hormonal issues except under the guidance of a qualified holistic medical practitioner.

Black Cohosh is widely known as a woman's herb to treat menstrual complaints. What is not widely known is its use as a muscle relaxer.

Black Cohosh has estrogen like qualities. It is used in women's formulas to normalize and regulate women's hormones, bring on delayed childbirth and menstruation, and help relieve menstrual stress and nervous tension.

Black Cohosh is a native American plant that grows in the deep shades of the eastern forest. It grows about 1 ½ feet tall, having leaves that resemble elm trees. When in bloom it produces a wand like stem that grows to 7 feet tall. The bloom does not have petals but a white stamen. It begins blooming around May and goes until September.

Do not use if pregnant or nursing without medical supervision.

CALENDULA

Calendula officinalis

Parts used: The petals and flower head

Anti-inflammatory, anti-fungal, antiseptic, wound healing, for skin irritations and burns, mucus membranes irritations, cell regeneration.

External uses:
Calendula is used in many skin creams and lotions. It is good as a skin cream for a silky complexion.

Calendula makes a soothing and gentle cream for treating cradle cap, diaper rash and skin irritations.

It is used in healing creams and salves for bruises, burns, sores, skin ulcers, infections and rashes.
Calendula not only helps with cell regeneration but is also antiseptic. Comfrey is well known for its cell regeneration, but can heal over an infection. Calendula acts as an antiseptic also, so reduces the chances of healing over an infection. Calendula is often combined with Comfrey.

Internal Uses:
Tinctures and teas are used to promote the draining of the lymph glands, inflammatory problems of the digestion system, stagnant liver problems, sluggish digestion, irregular or painful periods.

Harvest when the buds are just opening. Pick during the heat of the day when the resins will the strongest and the flowers have the lowest water content. You know that you have a good quality buds if they are sticky with resin.

Dried buds are best for tea: Fresh flowers are best for tinctures, salves, ointments and creams.

In cooler climates grow in full sun and it will bloom until first frost. In the south, and here in Texas it will not hold up to our summer heat. Start the seeds in July or early August for the fall and early spring. Flowers start in about 6 weeks after planting.

ECHINACEA

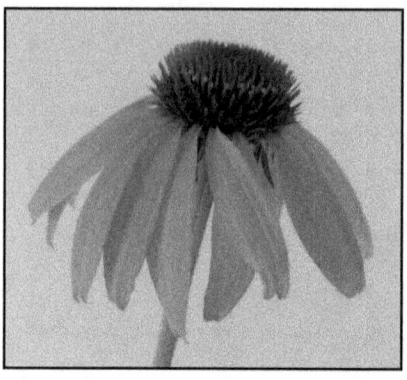

E. Purpurea, E. angustifolia, E. Pallida

Parts used: Roots, leaves, flowers, seeds

Immune system builder, increases antibody response, elevates interferon levels for fighting infections.

Wound infections, upper respiratory infections, mucus of the nose and sinus, throat infections and the root has a numbing effect on throat pain.

Echinacea is the most well studied herb in herbal remedies. Although daily doses of Echinacea will not prevent the flu or colds it will help shorten the length of the cold when a good quality is taken often enough.

Dosage: 1-2 ml (1/4 teaspoon) taken every 2 hours

Grows in full sun in the northern climates and partial shade here in Texas and the hot south.
Harvest flowers when they are fully opened, harvest the 3-4 years old roots in the late fall.

Grow from seed or the root.
Caution: Check with your medical professional if you have an auto immune disorder.

ELDER FLOWERS AND BERRIES

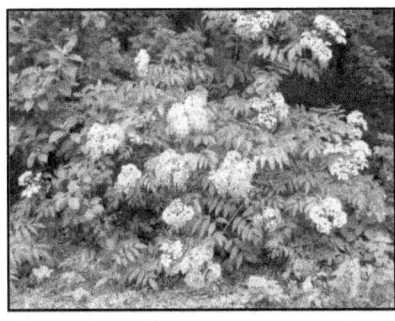

Sambucus nigra, S. cerulean, S. Canadensis

Parts used: flowers and berries, bark and leaves

Flowers: diaphoretic (induces sweating) combined with yarrow and peppermint to reduce fever by sweating.

Anti-Catarrhal of the nose (reduces excess mucus) combine with Peppermint, Echinacea and Yarrow.

Berries: immune stimulating and anti-viral for fighting colds, flu, herpes, shingles and upper respiratory infections. Combine with Echinacea

Leaves are used infused in ointments for bruises, sprains and wounds. Do not take internally, poisonous.

Bark: Purgative, emetic, diuretic

Elderberry is a common bush growing wild all over East Texas and other southern states. You will usually find it growing in the ditches or other wet areas. It is an old folk remedy at least 2500 years old.

Elder is easy to spot on the side of the road around June. During the month of June you can see the tiny white flowers that make up a big white umbrella shaped flower the size of a saucer.

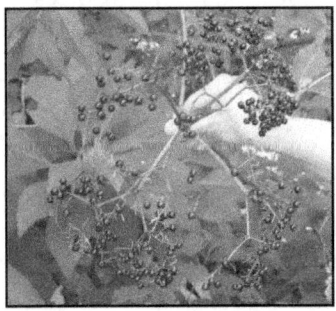

When these flowers turn into BB size berries the bushes seem to disappear into the woods and are much harder to spot.

The berries are ready to harvest when they turn black or blue (depending which species) in August or September, depending on the weather.

Don't try to pick the berries individually, just break off the whole umbrella shaped inflorescence. Have a basket handy underneath to catch any falling berries.

GARLIC

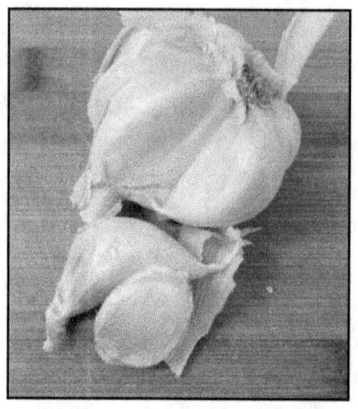

Allium sativum

Parts used: bulb

Anti-microbial, diaphoretic, cholagogue, hypotensive, anti-spasmodic

Used to treat colds, coughs, flu, diarrhea, infections, and heart health.

One of the most effective herbs well know around the world used as an internal and external antiseptic, antibacterial, and antimicrobial to treat infections. Garlic has been proven to fight off some antibiotic resistant bacteria. Garlic is used to treat worms in humans and animals.

Louis Pasteur documented garlic's antibacterial action in 1858. It was used in Africa by Albert Schweitzer to treat amoebic dysentery.

Modern research has confirmed that garlic can kill diarrhea causing Salmonella, Escherichia coli, Entamoeba histolytica and Giardia lablia.

Research also proves that taking garlic can prevent colds, lower blood pressure and cholesterol.

When using garlic as an antibiotic or antimicrobial mince or chop the garlic and let it set 10-15 minutes. The garlic cells must be ruptured to release two separate chemicals of the garlic, alliin and alliinase which then form a new compound called allicin.

For heart health extracts can be used if they are standardized to the key ingredient, allicin. Research suggests 4-8 mg a day to be effective.

Cautions: Because garlic can affect the platelets' ability to clots, avoid more than 4 cloves of garlic a day 10 days before surgery. Limit yourself to 4 cloves of garlic a day if taking anticoagulant medications. Consult your doctor if taking medications for HIV infections.

Growing conditions:

Grow in good garden soil, pointed end up, one inch deep, 6-12 inches apart.

In Texas and southern states, plant in the fall in full sun. In states where the ground freezes, plant in spring as soon as the ground thaws.

Harvest in spring when the leaves begin to fall over. For us that is usually late May or early June.

Save some bulbs to replant.

Store in peat moss.

Cutting back the flowers will produce bigger bulbs.

Caution: Discontinue use 10 days before surgery. Avoid more than 4 cloves a day if taking blood thinners.

GINGER

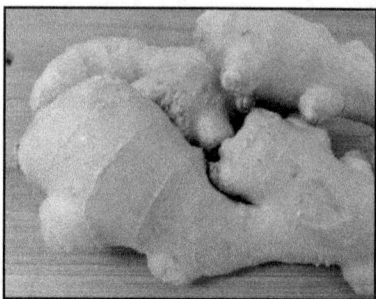

Zingiber officinale

Part used: rhizome

Used for morning sickness, motion sickness, nausea and vomiting, inflammation, coughs and colds.

Ginger is a stimulating herb and often used in herbal preparations as a carrier helping to move the other herbs through the body.

Ginger can be compared to Dramamine in its effectiveness for motion sickness and morning sickness and will not make you sleepy.
I use it when sinus drainage makes me nauseous.

For motion sickness, 1500 milligrams is recommended 30 minutes before travel. Ginger capsules can be used, or a 12 oz. glass of real Ginger Ale or Ginger tea. I prefer the Ginger candy. I keep it in my purse ready when I need it.

A hot foot bath of Ginger tea, may stop the onset of a cold, warm up cold feet and stop body pains. A cup of hot Ginger tea will increase circulation warming up toes, feet and hands and has virus killing compounds that will help ward of the cold or flu. A gargle of Ginger tea or Ginger tincture, will help a sore throat. A compress of Ginger tea placed over the throat can stop sore throat pain.

Ginger has been shown to reduce inflammation of arthritis but does not work as well as ibuprofen.

A Ginger compress over the lungs can help break up congestion. Ginger tea is my favorite for clearing up mucus.

The New England Journal of Medicine reports that Ginger reduces cholesterol, helps lower blood pressure and prevents internal blood clots.

The root of fresh Ginger is not boiled when making a tea, except when making Ginger Ale. The dried root is simmered.

Precautions: May cause heartburn, pregnant women should not take more than 1 gram of powdered Ginger a day, do not take large amounts of Ginger if you are taking blood thinners.

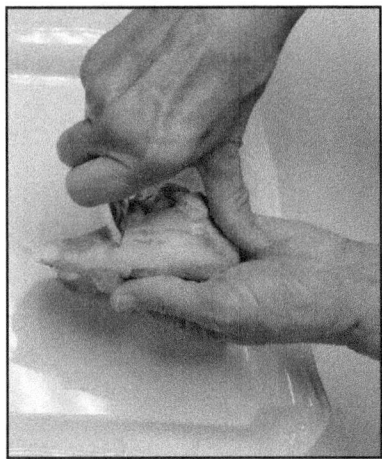

Use a spoon to peel ginger.

Growing Ginger:
Take a piece or fresh root that has at least 2 eyes. Plant in loose, rich soil with good drainage, barely covering the root and 12 inches apart. The temperature must be kept a minimum of 70°F constantly. The shoots should pop up in about 2 weeks. The roots or rhizomes should be ready to harvest in 9 months.

LEMON BALM

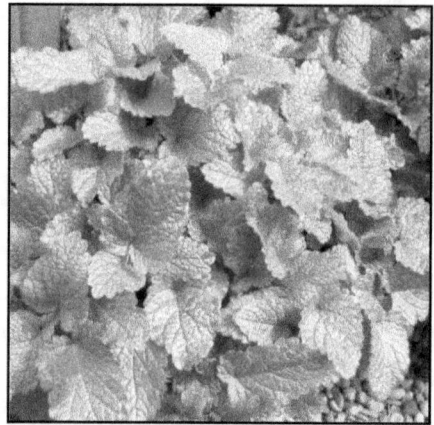

Melissa officinalis

Part used: leaves

Used for nervousness, insomnia, anxiety, herpes virus

Lemon Balm or Melissa is referred to as the gladdening herb.

Lemon Balm is the mildest tranquilizer to calm anxiety and stress, safe even for children. It gently relaxes the digestive muscles and has been used for centuries to relieve colic and digestion problems.

Lemon Balm is for any kind of nervous tension and stress.

It has be shown to calm heart spasms.

It is soothing for coughs and colds and PMS.

Caution using the essential oil of Lemon Balm (Melissa). Although it can be soothing to irritated skin, add very few drops to a carrier oil because it can also cause skin irritation. It is so expensive very few stores carry the product.

Teas, tinctures and extracts of Lemon Balm are safe to use.

It has antihistamine properties that will help with insect stings and helps heals wounds.

The extract of Lemon Balm is being used to decrease agitation in Alzheimer's patients and helps increase their memory.

It is often combined with hops and valerian to help with sleep and anxiety.

Studies show Lemon Balm lip ointment applied 3-4 times a day shortens and lessen the severity of herpes outbreaks. Lemon Balm combined with Licorice root is even more effective.

Lemon Balm may slightly interfere with thyroid hormones.

Lemon Balm is a perennial that likes moist but fast draining soil.

In Texas and the southern states it prefers some afternoon shade.

Harvest the leaves anytime during the growing season.

It will have better flavor before it blooms.

Keep the flowers cut back for more leaves.

LICORICE ROOT

Glycrrhiza glabra
Parts used: root

Used as an anti-viral, demulcent (makes things slippery and slimy), anti-inflammatory.

Use to soothe sore throats and inflamed throats, bronchial inflammations, stomach and bowel irritations and acts as a gentle laxative. Licorice Root low alcohol formulas will normally heal an ulcer within 24 hours. Research shows Licorice root is effective against the herpes simplex virus. Licorice Root is a specific remedy for adrenal exhaustion.

Because Licorice Root is 50 times sweeter than sugar so it is often combined with other herbs.

Growing conditions: Perennial, Full sun, alkaline soil, dryish soil
Hardy to 5°, grows 3-7 feet with mauve flowers.
Harvest in the fall of its 3rd or 4th year.

Caution: not to be used over a long period of time. It may cause water retention which would raise blood pressure. Do not use if you have high blood pressure, or heart or kidney problems without the guidance of a qualified health practitioner.

Licorice Root contains a compound called glycrrhizin which can deplete the body's potassium levels, causing water retention, which can lead to high blood pressure.

Deglycrrhizinated Licorice Root (DGL) has been developed for those who need to take Licorice Root for extended periods of time.

LOBELIA

Lobelia inflata
Parts used: top part

A low dose herb, only a few drops. Use to stop dry coughing and hacking, use as a bronchodilator to dilate the bronchial tubes, the main cough remedy for asthma, bronchitis, and whooping cough, use as an expectorant to thin mucus and help to cough it up.

A smooth muscle relaxer, use as liniments and plasters for sprains, muscle spasms and insect bites.

Use as a relaxant in case of trauma and hysteria.

Excessive doses will cause vomiting and sweating.

Growing conditions: Rich moist soil, a cool weather herb in Texas and the southern states. This herb will not do well if the soil temperature is over 70-75°f. Full sun in the northern states, or in the fall or winter in Texas, otherwise it may need partial shade.
Harvest the whole top once it flowers and there are a few developing seed capsules.

Alcohol, Vinegar, and Water will extract its properties.

Do not use if pregnant or nursing.

MULLEIN

Verbascum Thapsus
Parts used: leaves and flowers

Used as an expectorant (thins mucus), demulcent, anti-inflammatory, anti-spasmodic, and an astringent.

Mullein leaves are the number 1 choice for any respiratory problem. Mullein leaves may be used in cough medication to control coughs and helps to loosen mucus to move it out of the body.

Mullein leaf is combined with Lobelia and Echinacea for glandular imbalances.

The flowers are used to make the famous ear ache oil. The flowers are soaked in olive oil for 2-3 weeks, strained and poured into a dark brown bottle with a dropper dispenser. Warm the oil to body temperature and drop 3-4 drops of the Mullein flower infusion into each ear. Place a cotton ball into each ear to keep the oil from dripping out. Massage around the ear after applying the oil. This is repeated every few hours. A warm compress on the ear will make this more effective.
  Mullein flowers can be combined with Garlic for the same treatment.

This same oil can also be used for sunburn and rashes.

Mullein is considered safe except for the seeds. The seeds are considered toxic.

Mullein has pain easing properties that helps soothe nerve endings, reducing spasms associated with inflammation.

Growing conditions: Poor, sandy or gravely soil.
Mullein is a biennial. The first year it produces a rosette of long, flannel like, soft, fuzzy, lance-shaped leaves up to a foot long.
The second year it will grow a stalk up to 6 feet tall with small yellow flowers.
The leaves are harvested at the end of summer before they turn brown.
Mullein healing properties can be extracted in alcohol, vinegar and water.

Tea: 1-2 teaspoons of dried leaves and flowers to 1 cup of water, steeped for 10-15 minutes. Drink 3 times a day. Tincture: 1-4 ml (1/4 to 1 teaspoon 3 times a day.

NETTLES, STINGING NETTLES

Urtica dioica
Parts used: leaves, seeds. roots and young tops

Leaves are used for allergies and hay fever, arthritis, diuretic and eaten as a potherb for its calcium and other vitamins and minerals and as a tonic for the whole body.

Roots are used for Benign Prostatic Hyperplasia (BPH)

Yes this is the same weed that will sting you like a bee. The sting is caused from formic acid found on the underside of the leaves and the stalks.
The formic acid will be destroyed by drying, heating or mashing the leaves.

Nettles is used for hay fever and allergies while providing calcium and other nutrients for the growing pains of children and the achy bones of adults.

Freeze dried capsules are best for those taking Nettles for allergies.

Do not take close to bedtime as it is a diuretic and a stimulant.

Nettles is considered safe for everyone, except those who might be harvesting it without gloves. Ouch!!

Cautions: May cause interactions with medications for diabetes, high blood pressure, anxiety, or insomnia.

May cause impotence.

Growing conditions: Moist rich soil, semi- shade. Propagate from the runners in the spring or fall.

Harvest the young tops as a potherb for salads. Harvest the leaves for herbal remedies before they flower, harvest the roots in the fall.

MINTS

Mints are readily available, affordable and can be easily be grown at home. Their effectiveness has been proven in the marketplace.

Herbs are divided into Genus, and then further defined into species. While an herb may be in the same Genus, the specific species may have different properties.

Mints are well known in the kitchen and deserve a healthy respect in your herbal remedy kit.

Mints are divided into 3 groups, cooking, healing, and decoration. All mints are refreshing and cooling. All mints have square stems. Most of them are perennials, and if not killed by a hard freeze or lack of water are very invasive and will spread by their roots. Control mint spreading in your garden by planting in pots or in a bottomless container at least 10 " deep. Different mints will interbreed. Keep the flowers pinched off and different mint plants as far away from each other as you can. When you purchase mints at the nursery, rub the leaves to check the aroma.

Mints originally came from Europe and Asia. Mint naturalized in North America by the immigrants settling the country. Most mints are hardy to zone 5. It will grow in sun or shade with plenty of water. If you live in the southwest, like Texas, I can tell you from experience, spearmint will grow in full sun if given plenty of water. Peppermint may need a little afternoon shade.

Do not buy mint seeds. The only way to get the mint you really want is to propagate from cuttings or layering.

PEPPERMINT

Mentha piperita

The most well know mint is Peppermint. This is the mint used medically and in most of your candies, breath mints and treats. Peppermint tea is a well known remedy for indigestion, cramps and headaches. The essential oil of Peppermint is also well known as a remedy for toothaches and muscle soreness. Peppermint is the herb you would use with chocolate, coffee and candies.

The menthol in Peppermint is well known as a digestive aid. Everyone has inhaled menthol for respiratory problems. Menthol is the main ingredient in Vicks Rub. The vapors from Vicks Rub or other ointments containing menthol are rubbed on the neck and chest to help relieve a stuffy nose.

Peppermint grows closer to the ground, has smaller leaves than spearmint. It requires more shade and more water than Spearmint.

Peppermint Tea
1 cup of boiling water
1 teaspoon dried Peppermint leaves or Peppermint tea bag, or 6-8 fresh leaves
Pour boiling water over the Peppermint, steep for 10 minutes. Strain and take a sip. Pucker up and suck air through your lips. You will notice the cool effect from the menthol in the Peppermint tea.

A cup of warm Peppermint tea will thin mucus and loosen phlegm and help relieve a stuffy nose. Peppermint tea is good as a digestive aid.

Peppermint for Headaches

Peppermint Headache Compress, good for sinus or tension headache
Add ice cubes to prepared peppermint tea. Wet washcloth in cold tea and apply to forehead.

Peppermint Tea Foot Soak
Pour 1 quart of boiling water over a handful for Peppermint leaves and let steep for 5 minutes. Use warm in the winter to stimulate circulation for colds and the flu. Add ice to make a soak for hot tired feet.

Peppermint for Itchy Eyes

Soak Peppermint tea bags in hot water for 30 minutes. Cool and place on eyes.

Cautions: Do not use Peppermint if you have a Hiatal hernia or heartburn.

Caution using essential oil of Peppermint on children under 3.

SPEARMINT AND OTHER MINTS

Spearmint: Mentha: spicata, or viridis

Even though the Spearmint is cool and refreshing, you will notice there is no menthol.

Spearmint, fruity mints and curly mints contain no menthol and are generally used for cooking. Spearmint can be used instead of Peppermint on children for inflammation and as an antiseptic.

Spearmint is what you would use to make a mint cucumber sauce or use with lamb. Spearmint is the mint for Greek, Arabic, North African, Indian and Middle Eastern dishes. Spearmint is the mint for Mint Juleps, Mojitos, and other drinks.

Mint Juleps, Mojitos and Wriggly Spearmint gum! No wonder the 16 century herbalist wrote, "The smell rejoiceth the heart of man ". And, I might add, it is the mint for lovers.

The aroma of Spearmint opens and releases emotional blocks and brings about a feeling of well being and balance.

Spearmint is cooling and refreshing in the summer heat. Just smelling the aroma seems to help cool you off.

Spearmint will grow in full sun even in Texas and get maybe 2 feet tall. I have seen some varieties given more shade and more water get 3-4 feet tall. Giving the spearmint a little shade and more water will give you bigger leaves. Cut it often to keep it shorter and keep it from looking weedy and scraggly. Keeping it cut back will force the stems to branch out and make the plants look lush and healthy, and of course give you more leaves.

Spearmint is hardy to zone 5. It is a kind of a dark lime green, which is why I suppose it goes so well with limes and lemons. It has rough, jagged pointed leaves that grow up a square stem. The younger the stem the closer together the leaves will be. If you let your spearmint go too long without cutting it back, the leaves will grow further and further apart. If you can't drink that many Mojitos or mint tea or lemonade tie it up in little bundles and hang them around the house or on the porch for that little bit of fragrant cottage ambience. Or, of course, you might also be accused of being a witch.

Spearmint is invasive and will take over your garden. If you don't' absolutely love spearmint and think the more the better either grow it in a pot, or put a barrier of some sort around it at least 10" deep. It will grow through mulch and rocks.

Using spearmint in any of your bath or body products will be restorative and stimulating, according to Jeanne Rose, who also adds that spearmint feels good and strengthens the nerves and muscles. She also includes mint as one the 6 best herbs for cosmetics. Rose, Thyme, Comfrey, Mint, Lavender and Rosemary. Jeanne Rose's Herbal Body Book

Simple ways to use Spearmint
Bruise 1 cup of mint leaves, add to a half gallon pitcher (2 qt.), fill with water and refrigerate. After it is chilled, strain and serve over ice. You could also use this to rinse off your face or your body to cool off.
Add a sprig to your lemonade or ice tea.

Apple mint, Pineapple Mint, and the other fruity mints are mostly used for garnishing drinks and flavoring things like cottage cheese.

SLIPPERY ELM

Ulmus fulva, or rubra
Parts used: the inner bark

Medical Properties: Occasional heartburn, coughs, sore throat, itchy inflamed skin, irritations of the mouth, throat, stomach and intestines.

Slippery Elm is one of the few herbs actually approved by the FDA. It is not only a great healing herb for irritations internally or externally it is also a food. It has about the same nutrition as oatmeal. It is used as a gruel or porridge for those recovering from illness such as diarrhea, and those with gastro-intestinal illnesses.

George Washington and his troops survived on Slippery Elm Porridge for 12 days during the American Revolution.

Slippery Elm powder becomes mucilaginous or slimy when it becomes in contact with water. It soothes irritated throats as well as irritated stomachs internally and can be made into a paste to be applied externally to soothe itchy, irritated, inflamed skin.

It can be drunk as a tea, or sucked on as lozenges.

Tea: Pour 1 cup of boiling water over 1-2 teaspoon of the powdered bark and steep for 5 minutes. Drink 2-3 times per day as need.

Lozenges: As needed

Externally: Mix 2 tablespoons of the powdered bark with 1/4 cup of water to make a paste. Apply to itchy inflamed skin for 20-30 minutes. Reapply as needed.

Caution: Do not use on open wounds. Do not use if you have bile duct obstruction or gallstones.

May slow the absorption of medications, use 1 hour before taking medication or several hours after taking medication.

ST. JOHN'S WORT

Hypericum perforatum L.
Parts used: aerial parts

Used to treat minor depression, sciatica and other nerve pain, and anxiety. Salves and lotions are used to treat mild burns, sunburns and bruises.

Research has proven that is effective to treat mild depression but not major depression.

The oil of St. John's Wort is used as an anti-inflammatory, and is used to treat mild burns, bruises, and skin injuries.

The flowers and tops are harvested when the buds are ripe and the flowers just open.

Growing conditions: Grows in average garden soil, in full sun. It likes acid conditions and good drainage.

VALERIAN

Valeriana officinalis
Parts used: Rhizome, stolons, and roots

Valerian Root is used as a sleep aid, muscle relaxer, for anxiety and nervousness.

It has a well deserved reputation as a sleep aid. While sleeping pills effect REM, Valerian does not. It will not affect your dreams like sleeping pills and is considered completely safe and non habit forming.

It can be safely used for muscle cramping, uterine cramps and intestinal colic.

Valerian is used worldwide and was validated by WHO as a relaxing remedy to treat cardiovascular problems. It is combined with Hawthorn Berry to treat irregular heartbeat and high blood pressure.

Valerian works even better when combined with other herbs. It is combined with Skullcap for tension and anxiety.

A combinations of Hops or Passionflower with Valerian Root is better for sleep.
Combine Valerian with Chamomile or Lavender for nervous indigestion, and Black Haw or Cramp Bark for muscular cramps.

Valerian Root must be taken in large enough doses to be effective. The most popular way to take Valerian Root is by tincture. Start with ½ to 1 teaspoon. Although it is very unlikely that you could overdose on Valerian, it is better to take 1 teaspoon several times in a short period of time, rather than take a larger dose.

You know you have taken too much if your legs start feeling rubbery.

There are a small amount of people that Valerian Root has the opposite effect. It will make them feel irritated and wired up. If you have never taken Valerian Root it would be wise to start with a small dose and see how you feel before taking more.

Growing conditions: Partial shade to full sun and moist, rich soil.

About the AUTHOR

Carolyn Gibson LMT, MTI CE Provider, and Family Herbalist has been a registered massage therapist since 1996. She fell in love with herbs in the early 70's and has been growing herbs, studying, using and making herbal remedies since that time.

She and her husband Gerald Gibson are the owners of Dogwood Gardens Organic Farm, certified organic since 1991.

They began growing medical herbs and now grow Wheatgrass only.

Contact Carolyn at www.FamilyGuidetoHerbs.com
903 833 1024
CarolynGibson1951@gmail.com

Other Books by Carolyn Gibson
On Amazon: and website

How to be a Good Wife
Trigger Point Made Easy
Myths, Mysteries and Benefits of Herbs and Essential Oils
(Herbs and Essential Oils for Texas Massage Therapist)

Books on Kindle:

All About Wheatgrass
How to Be a Good Wife
Myths, Mysteries and Benefits of Herbs and Essential Oils
Unique DIY Centerpieces